Jaw Recovery Playbook

Offense Playbook

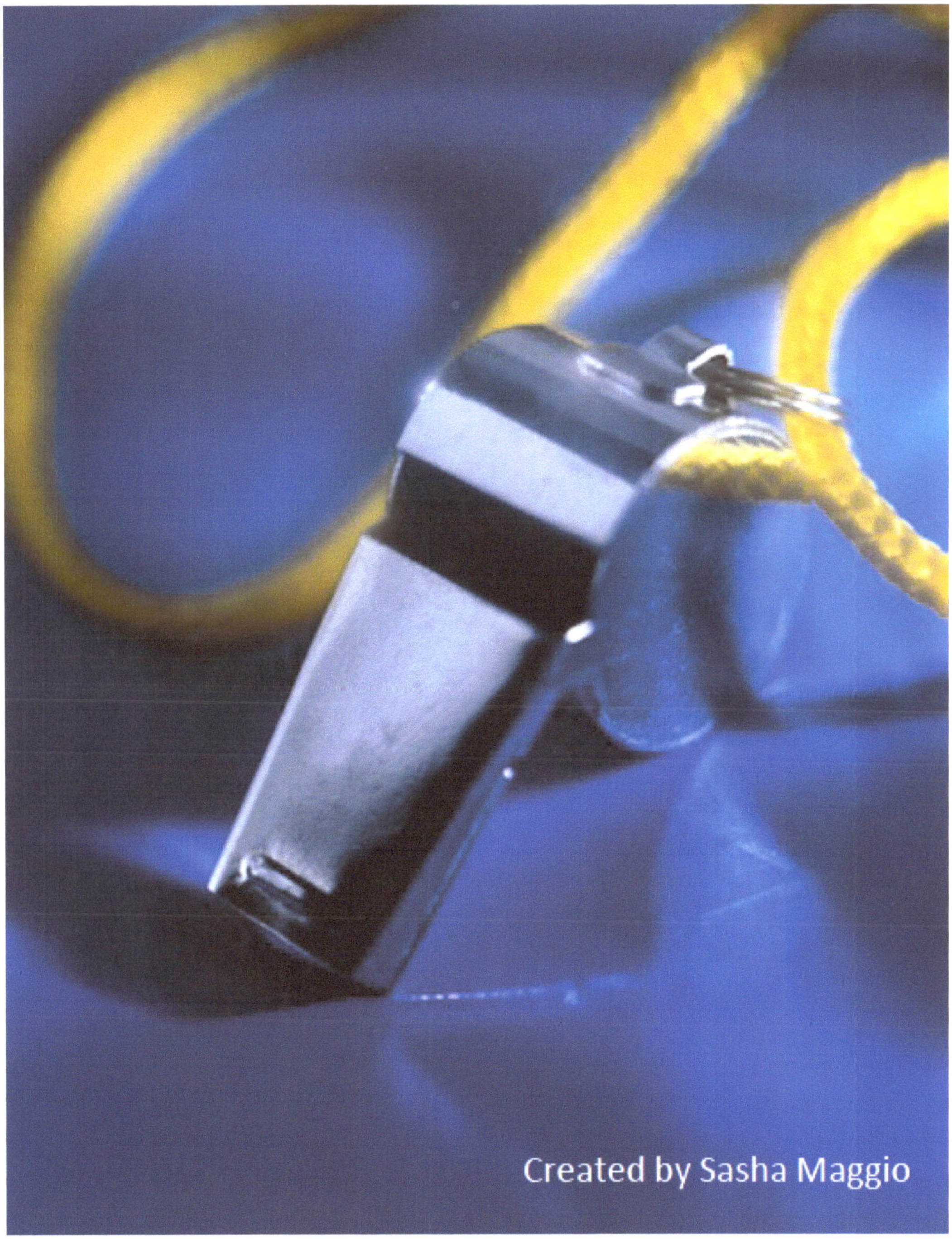

Created by Sasha Maggio

© 2011. Sasha Maggio. All Rights Reserved.
(Updated © 2014. Sasha Maggio. All Rights Reserved.)
No portion of this book or the Jaw Recovery Playbook System, including the recipes, website, name, themes, likeness, content or ideas may be reproduced or transmitted in any form without the expressed written consent of Sasha Maggio. Contact the Jaw Recovery Playbook for permission.

Registered or patented products such as Invisalign, Trace Minerals, Crest, BareMinerals, Aveeno, Neutrogena, True Citrus, Truvia/Stevia, Blistex, or any other brand/product, are listed with a note and/or link to the patent-holder, company, or manufacturer website. Any brands listed are for demonstrative purposes only and do not denote sponsorship, endorsement, or support of any kind.

Regarding Images Used in the Jaw Recovery Playbook: Offense Playbook by Sasha Maggio

Images created by Sasha Maggio for the Jaw Recovery Playbook are labeled as such.

Images of specific brand products are labeled to show the source of the images with links provided for reader use. The use of these images is for example only and does not reflect any form of support or endorsement by the companies or manufacturers depicted.

All non-labeled images are from Microsoft Office ClipArt and images, available freely at www.office.microsoft.com, used in accordance with the Microsoft Office Images guidelines. The use of these images does not, in any way, reflect the opinions, endorsement, or support of Microsoft or www.office.microsoft.com. The images from Microsoft Office are for decorative effect only.

The original content created by Sasha Maggio serves as the primary value of the Jaw Recovery Playbook website and playbooks. Original content includes, but is not limited to, all written text, photographs and images created by Sasha Maggio, website design components, and original themes and/or ideas presented throughout the Jaw Recovery Playbook resources and website.

Contact information is available at www.JawRecoveryPlaybook.com for questions, comments, and written permission for reproduction or use of any portion of the original content.

When in doubt ~ ASK

Legal Disclaimer

I am not now, nor have I ever been a medical doctor, nutritionist, registered dietician, nurse, dentist, or any other medical professional; at least not at the time of this writing. My education is in psychology, with pre-professional science courses, and I have conducted ~~hundreds~~ thousands of hours of independent research and studying in physical fitness, nutrition, biology, anatomy and physiology, neurology, and other fields that hold personal relevance.

The information provided throughout the Jaw Recovery Playbook system, including this Playbook, other Playbooks, and the online content, is intended for personal use only. The information is not intended to diagnose, treat, or otherwise replace actual medical care. If something in the content and Playbooks resembles symptoms you are experiencing, consult your primary doctor, surgeon, orthodontist, dentist, or other healthcare professional involved in your current preventative and active care.

The information here is the result of hundreds of hours of independent research through scientific, scholarly, psychological, and sociological sources for the purpose of improving my own efforts to manage my jaw surgery experience, recovery process, and related health. The information is accurate and up to date, to the best of my knowledge, and will be updated if new publications contradict or enhance what I have presented here.

This information is not a substitute for proper healthcare but can inform patients and caregivers of many aspects of the jaw surgery process and improve efforts to prepare effectively.

Feel free to contact me at JawRecoveryPlaybook@gmail.com to inform of any mistakes found; I am, after all, only human. If you find a mistake or inaccuracy in the content, please provide a link to the resource you are using for comparison so that I can correct as needed and cite appropriately.

S.M.

http://www.jawrecoveryplaybook.com/legal/

Dedicated to...

The Jaw Recovery Playbook System, composed of the website, Playbooks, and other original content, are the result of over two years of diligent effort. When studying something that is not school-related or work-related, the greatest challenge one typically faces is staying motivated. I could not have continued with such passionate drive if it weren't for the support of my family and husband, always encouraging me to do the best I can and reassuring me that the knowledge I acquired for my own recovery was something I simply HAD to share with others.

The incredible support and feedback I received from my orthodontist, Dr. Allen Garai, and his team at Garai Orthodontic Specialists in Vienna, VA, nurtured my drive to do more with my Playbook System. I could not have asked for better care than I received at Garai Orthodontic Specialists - choosing them for my care was definitely the best decision I made during my treatment process!

I also could not have completed the Playbook System without the support I received from my oral & maxillofacial surgeons, the staff, and other technicians at Walter Reed National Military Medical Center in Bethesda, MD. The Oral & Maxillofacial Surgery department at Walter Reed was a great fit for me, and my treatment, despite the occasionally bumpy road throughout the initial treatment process while I approached "surgery-ready." My surgeons took the time to answer my questions and the entire department was nothing short of amazing when it came to personalizing my care. Their positive feedback throughout my recovery also fueled my desire to learn more and bring my Jaw Recovery Playbook System to a unique level.

The Jaw Recovery Playbook System would not exist if it were not for the important roles you each played in my treatment and recovery, and I am forever grateful for the experience to meet and work with all of you!

-Sasha

About the Author

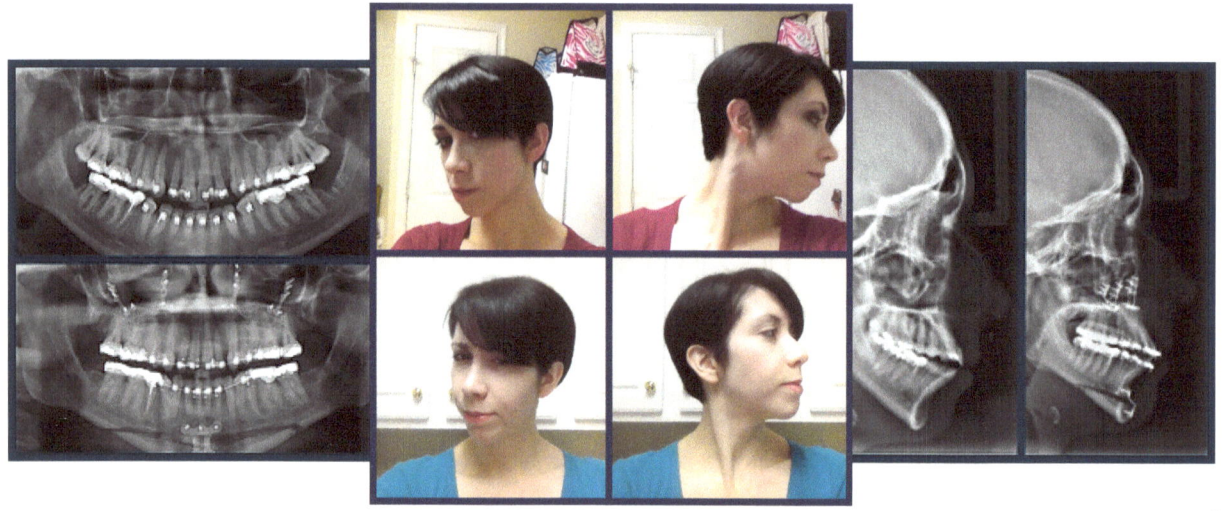

© Photos by Sasha Maggio
December 12, 2011, the day before surgery (top).
January 2012, 6 weeks after surgery (bottom).

Sasha Maggio is a professional business writer specializing in copywriting for marketing, advertisements, product catalogs, and website content. She holds a B.A. in Psychology, with a Minor in Japanese, from the University of Hawaii and an M.A. in Forensic Psychology.

After wearing braces as a teenager, Sasha noticed her open-bite slowly returning over the course of 10 years. Consulting an orthodontist, she was informed she would need jaw surgery and standard braces to repair the problem. As she prepared for her own surgery, Sasha noticed a trend in the available information and resources for jaw surgery patients. The majority of information widely available for patients fell short of her expectations for a healthy, relatively easy recovery after surgery. With no quality resources in sight, she created the Jaw Recovery Playbook; a website and resource for jaw surgery patients, caregivers, and surgeons to improve treatment experiences for all.

In December 2011, Sasha underwent upper and lower jaw surgery, with revision in March 2013. Since developing the Jaw Recovery Playbook, she has regularly helped jaw surgery patients across the globe as they prepare for their jaw surgeries.

Sasha lives "wherever the Army sends us" with her husband, a career Army Officer, and their three dogs: Jake, Zoya, and Atom.

Forward

Part guidebook, part memoir of my own jaw surgery and recovery experience, the Jaw Recovery Playbook was designed to help other jaw surgery patients, their families and caregivers, and providers (surgeons, orthodontists, dentists, etc.) understand, explain, and prepare for the complete jaw surgery experience. To aid comprehension, I have divided the information into different resources geared toward helping specific people at specific times.

The Offense Playbook was designed for the jaw surgery patient, while the Offensive Coordinator Playbook was designed for the patient's providers. "Providers" is a broad term I use to refer to everyone involved in the patient's healthcare from their general dentist to their orthodontist to their oral & maxillofacial surgeon and/or surgical team. The Defense Playbook is geared toward helping family members, partners, friends, and loved ones understand what the patient is going through, what the patient needs, and how they can help as part of the patient's overall Team.

The Recipe Playbook contains the recipes I used during my jaw surgery recovery, along with information to help guide recipe creation for patients who feel up to the creative task. Since the jaw surgery recovery process differs for patients, I also included tips for easier nutrition and eating whether the jaws can open or are bound shut with bands.

The Game Day Playbook helps the patient mentally and physically prepare for their surgery date and I combined the Game Day Playbook with the Recovery Playbook, which addresses common struggles and can serve as a guide to help the patient improve his or her own recovery process. It made sense to keep these two together since Game Day is but one small part of the jaw surgery experience and it's the first step in the recovery process.

While the examples mentioned are often my own or from interaction with patients that I have helped, thus anecdotal, I have refrained from naming specific patients that have sought my help but may include their struggles as general examples - using phrases such as "many jaw surgery patients" "some jaw surgery patients" or "common problems/struggles/issues for jaw surgery patients are..." This is to maintain their privacy, but mentioned here to explain where the statements come from.

When I faced the very idea of jaw surgery, before ever consulting a surgeon and before my braces were applied (for the second time in my life), I was absolutely terrified. I submitted my referral to consult a surgeon and while I waited for my insurance company to process that referral I browsed the internet for information. That was when I first realized that resources for jaw surgery patients were considerably limited.

There are countless jaw surgery blogs by other patients, but many follow one of four trends:

1. They journal the entire pre-surgery and recovery experience in (at least moderate) detail, including pictures, but provide little or no real guidance regarding the healing process beyond one or two recipes and their self-reported feelings and frustrations throughout.

2. They journal in pseudo-detail, usually without pictures, and provide no real guidance beyond their own thoughts, experiences and struggles.

3. They journal infrequently, providing a little insight into their experience but with such large time gaps between blog posts that it's difficult to maintain interest in their experience and they leave readers with no hope for useful information.

4. They start to journal in detail, then seem to drop out of sight after surgery – which is usually either because recovery was more difficult than they expected and they didn't want to share anymore, or their recovery was easier than expected so they didn't feel motivated to keep sharing.

Faced with this realization, I knew I was on my own. I spent 16 months leading up to surgery researching. Among other things, I researched nutrition, anatomy & physiology to better understand healing, patient psychology, and the procedures I was to undergo. The procedures are quite scary when you know little about them, and I have to admit, they can still be quite scary even if you know a lot about them. The information was important to me, and knowing gave me greater confidence in the surgical team and potential for success.

I underwent surgery on 13 December 2011 and I anticipated a difficult recovery. I expected to be miserable. I expected to crave real food. I expected to be bored. I expected pain, terrible swelling, exhaustion, and just all around misery. What I got, however, was completely different and entirely unexpected. While the first day home was a little difficult because the recipes I had planned to use proved to be less-than-friendly with my syringes, the overall recovery experience was extremely easy. I believe that easy recovery was the direct result of diligent focus on maintaining nutrition, staying hydrated, resting as needed but avoiding sleep except at night, and the support of my own Team.

As other patients found my personal blog and read my notes on jaw surgery recovery, watched my videos, and saw my pictures, they began contacting me for guidance and support. Following the guidance I offered and making adjustments where needed, dozens of patients have been able to turn their miserable recoveries around and end strong and pleased with the experience. Other patients have contacted me in advance and managed to survive their recoveries with ease from the beginning. Patients of all ages, from all over the world, have been using my Jaw Recovery Playbook before it even existed, and their success has made me very proud of them, but also honored to have been trusted for help and allowed to be part of their surgery and recovery experiences too.

After surgery, I decided to build the Jaw Recovery Playbook website, which faced its own struggles as I recovered from post-surgery anemia and managed my way back into regular everyday life with work, family, and responsibilities. I continued working on the individual Playbooks and it took over a year but I am very happy that I now have a more organized way to help all the patients that contact me...and there are MANY!

I could have simply healed and moved on with my life, but the responses from those I've helped and the encouragement from others who witnessed my recovery showed me I could not simply forget this information or let it go to waste.

Jaw surgery is a very special experience that most people will never understand. Patients that undergo surgery for corrective reasons (and possibly cosmetic) truly appreciate the life-changing nature of this experience and every patient that I know is pleased they went through with it.
Jaw surgery doesn't have to be scary. Recovery doesn't have to be a struggle. You can make the choice and control it - and the Jaw Recovery Playbook System can help!

For free resources and information, frequently asked questions, videos, contact information, and more - visit www.JawRecoveryPlaybook.com

The other Playbooks are available through iBooks, Kindle, and as PDF downloads with PayPal check out on the website.

Thank you for trying to improve your jaw surgery experience and trusting the Jaw Recovery Playbook to help. Encourage those involved in your recovery to consider the resources I have compiled for them as well, to improve the way you all work together for a common goal - the patient's surgery, recovery, and return to normal life with little difficulty.

~Sasha Maggio

Note: When mentioning pronouns for orthodontists, surgeons, and others throughout the Playbook I use "he" and "she" interchangeably but often default to "he" because my providers were all male.

Contents

1. Introduction
   - Jaw Surgery Basics
   - You are the Quarterback & Team Captain
2. So I'm having Jaw Surgery… Now What?
   - How soon is 'too soon' to prepare?
   - Manage Your Own Treatment
3. Skincare Before & After Surgery
4. Basic Nutrition
   - Macronutrients
   - Micronutrients
   - Calculate Your Dietary Needs
   - Menu Planning
   - Better Habits for Better Recovery
5. Patient Psychology
   - Mentally Preparing for Jaw Surgery
   - Finding Control
   - Dealing with Others
   - Expectation Management
6. What do I do if…?
   - My orthodontist said I'm ready BUT my surgeon said I'm not…
   - My Timeline Keeps Changing!
   - I'm sick of this!
7. Jaw Recovery Playbook
8. Where do I go next?
9. Glossary
10. Bibliography & Resources

1
Introduction

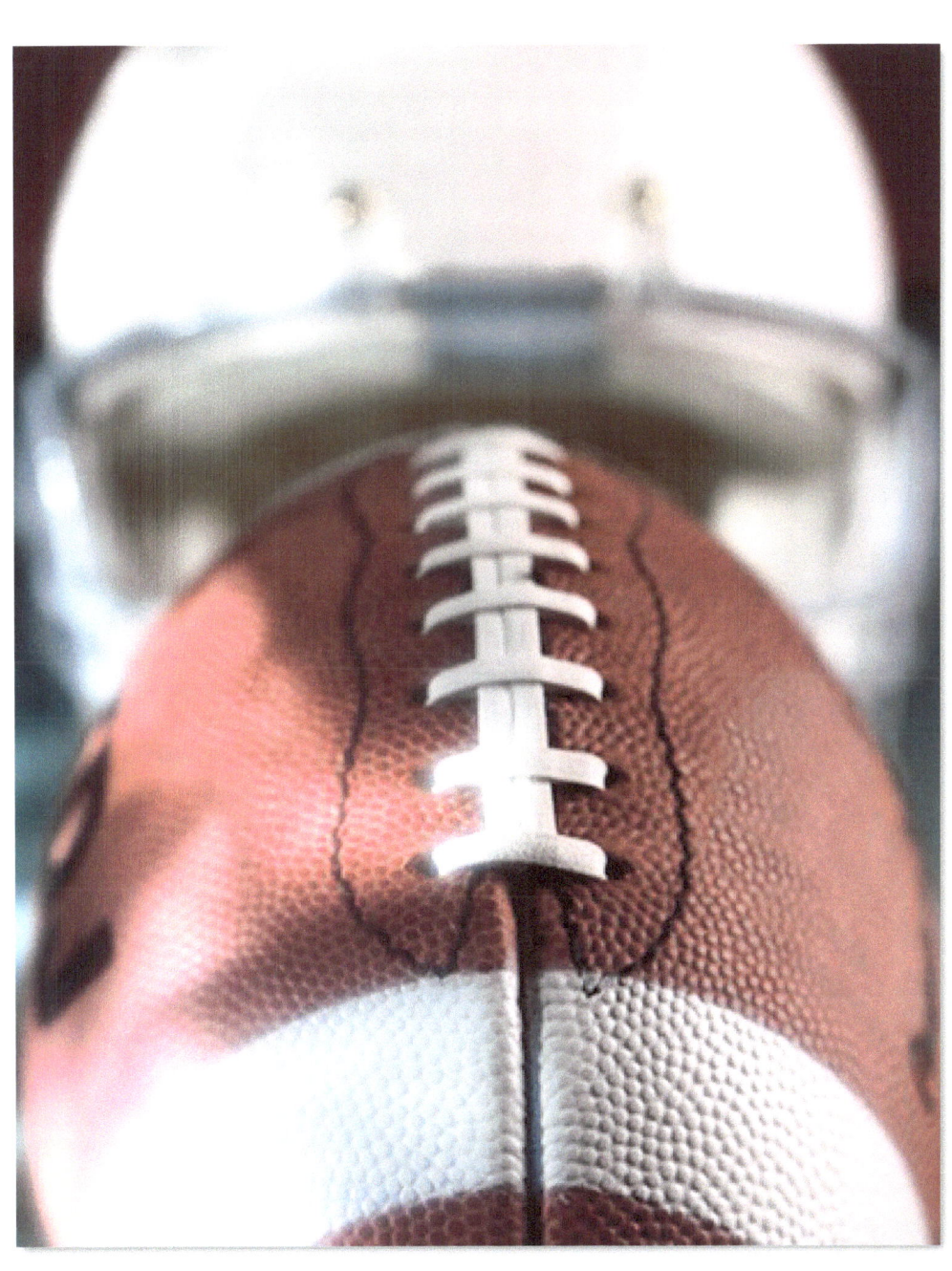

Jaw Surgery Basics

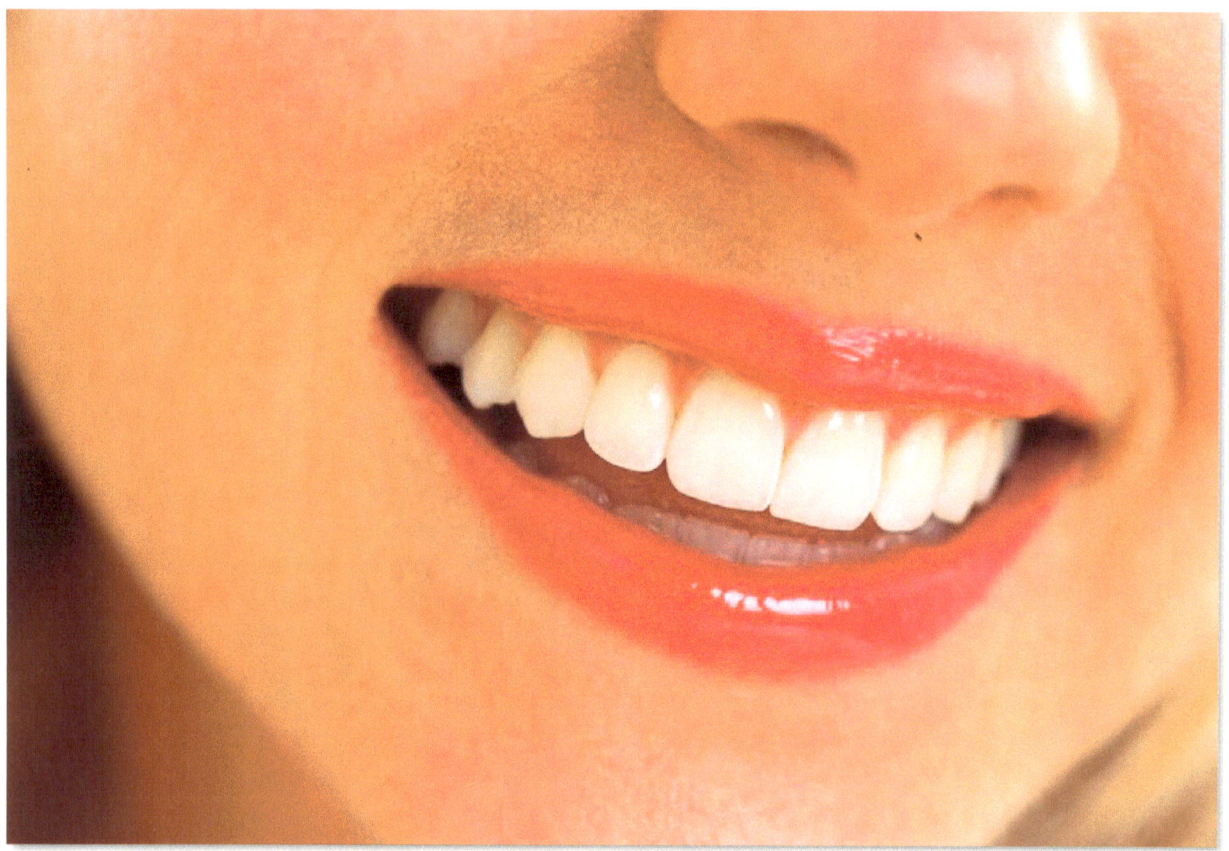

One of the first questions that runs through many patients' minds is, "why me?" We all wonder why. Why do I need jaw surgery when so-and-so has the same problem and she didn't need jaw surgery? Why can't I just have braces? And if I need surgery then why do I need braces?

I consulted two orthodontists before I accepted my fate as a jaw surgery patient. The first orthodontist did not present the situation very well! I felt he couldn't possibly be serious; I mean, that top jaw is permanently attached to my face. It wasn't going anywhere!

I feared that if the bottom jaw was operated on, it would make my TMJ issues worse. The issues were tolerable most of the time, but they began when I had braces as a teenager. The rubber bands, at that time, put so much pressure on the joints that I began experiencing bouts of lock-jaw, and usually during lunch at school. I would go to bite into a sandwich or other food and my jaw would suddenly lock. It would be about a half-inch open and I'd be unable to open or close any further. This would usually last a few moments before my attempts to come out of the locked position would take, but those occasional experiences over the 10 years since I wore braces were sufficient to cause some apprehension when thinking of possible lower-jaw surgery, and as I mentioned before, I didn't think upper-jaw surgery was even possible.

It was about a year later that I consulted my orthodontist, after a very careful selection process. I wanted to make sure that who I saw next for a consult was not only qualified, but had a long history or excellent service in his field. When he explained that jaw surgery was necessary to fix my problem-bite, I believed him. He took the time to explain what was needed, what the potential timeline would look like, and what to expect, at least on a basic level. He gave me a referral, outlined all the pricing for braces and what my options were, and he presented everything in a professional way that made me feel like he was treating me as an adult and a valuable potential-patient, not just some random person in for the free consult with no intentions of coming back.

I admit, when I learned I couldn't have something like Invisalign* or lingual braces* (notes at end of section), I was disappointed but the possibility of an actual permanent fix to my open-bite was appealing enough to make it worth trying.

I had made the decision to at least consult with an oral surgeon to see what I should expect, and possibly any alternatives. In my case, my lower jaw didn't grow completely, so it always felt as if it was set back too much. I described it to my first jaw surgery Resident as feeling like I was always pushing my chin toward my chest or neck. So I could feel what the problem was but I thought it was a habit that I had to break, like nail biting, as if I had grown into habitually pulling my chin down and back. I knew I had an issue with tongue-thrust because I had speech therapy as a kid (third grade). I was taught to pronounce my /s/ and /th/ sounds properly but no training to improve my chewing and swallowing so I continued with a significant amount of problem chewing, swallowing, and talking behaviors.

I thought that my problem was an open-bite caused by my upper teeth pointing forward too much. Tongue-thrust would aggravate this, but throughout that series of consultations I learned something I had never heard before. I learned that tongue-thrust is not always the actual underlying issue. In my case, the issue was from the malformed jaws. If the jaws were aligned properly, my tongue would rest in its proper place and I would have greater control over naturally chewing, swallowing, and speaking without the thrust motion.

I also learned that the fact that my lower jaw was shorter than it should be, in a sense, moving the lower jaw forward with a Bilateral Sagittal Split-Osteotomy (or BSSO) and adjusting the size, shape, and angle of the upper jaw with a 3-piece Le Fort I procedure would permanently fix my alignment issues which would, in turn, help fix the tongue-thrust behavior issue. Although it's scary, this was the first time the situation seemed positive.

I hadn't known how common these surgeries were until discussing it with the surgeons. Apparently that's common too, as many patients don't realize how many people actually undergo these and similar jaw surgery procedures.

So who needs jaw surgery?

Typically speaking, jaw surgery is performed on patients whose occlusion (the way their teeth come together) cannot be fixed by braces alone. This is something the orthodontist and surgeons will recognize once they see the X-rays, impressions, and take measurements of the face and head. There are some instances when surgery may be a possibility but the providers aren't certain until orthodontic treatment begins.

Jaw surgery is not cheap. It's not mindlessly offered to all patients. It's not meant to scare them or to make their treatment process more difficult. If your orthodontist believes jaw surgery is necessary, he will refer you to an oral & maxillofacial surgeon for a consultation to be sure. This referral and the surgeon's input is essential to treatment planning because if you have only braces, your treatment takes a standard route but if you need jaw surgery your teeth are not moved in the same fashion.

How do braces differ for jaw surgery patients?

The braces will vary depending on the problem and the solution. For example, in my case with an open-bite, my braces pulled my teeth open even more, making the open-bite worse than it had ever been. This was so that at the time of surgery, when the surgeon repositioned my upper jaw, the upper teeth were in the right places to line up in their NEW position with the lower jaw. I was aware that this would happen and it wasn't the easiest thing to deal with because it was considerably more uncomfortable to eat, chew, speak, and smile. It increased my self-consciousness with all of those activities as well, but **I knew it would only be temporary** so I managed to push through my discomfort with a positive attitude.

Another patient that consulted me had an unfortunate experience in which her orthodontist was not informed of what to do for jaw surgery preparation. After a year in braces with her teeth straightened and pulled back for an improved alignment, but still with an open-bite, the surgeon saw her and sent her back to the orthodontist to almost completely reverse everything they had done throughout that first year. Her teeth had to be pulled forward and open the bite more. This was very frustrating for her but demonstrates the importance of taking control of your own treatment and making sure that your surgeon and orthodontist are clearly communicating. This is discussed later in the Patient Psychology chapter.

Another variation with braces for surgery depends on the procedures. In my case, with a 3-piece Le Fort I, my orthodontist had to create gaps on either side of the upper incisors (the front teeth). This was done using a tiny spring, smaller than the spring in a pen but similar in appearance. The spring was placed on my archwire in-between the brackets on the teeth where the gaps had to be made. For me, this was between the canines and the lateral incisors, I believe. It wasn't painful, but the gaps were big! About 2mm or a little wider so it was significant, and very obvious any time I opened my mouth, adding to my self-consciousness but again, **you learn to manage by focusing on the**

end-result and not focusing completely on the process.

These gaps are for the surgeon to safely segment the upper jaw in order to reshape it. Since I was receiving a 3-piece Le Fort I, the upper jaw was segmented into three pieces, with the cuts almost like a Y-shape along the palate. The upper jaw stays connected with the soft tissue, and relatively "together," throughout the surgery, so do not let this stir up panic. It allows the surgeon to widen or shrink the shape of the upper jaw in order to improve its fit and functionality.

These gaps are not made until the patient is near surgery-ready so you should not expect to see them for a long time and some patients never have them because they're not necessary for that patient's procedures.

Surgical Wires and Surgical Hooks

When the patient is finally near surgery-ready, the orthodontist will swap the archwires for surgical wires which are basically just another type of archwire. Surgical hooks will also be added. In my case, some of my brackets contained hooks for surgery while additional hooks were clamped along the archwires at specific locations.

With the 3-piece Le Fort I, the wires had to be cut in order to accommodate the reshaping, so when I woke up after surgery there were two spots were the gaps between my teeth had been that now had the cut ends of the archwire slightly over-lapping. The gaps were still present, but reduced in size. They are closed by the orthodontist after recovery while he completes the orthodontic treatment process.

The surgical hooks are used to ensure proper alignment of the upper and lower jaws during surgery. Basically, the surgeon uses the hooks to make sure that when they attach brackets and stitch up the fleshy soft tissue, the teeth and jaws are properly aligned so the patient heals well. The hooks are also used to bind the teeth shut with a ton of rubber bands. Typically, the patient is bound shut like that for a day or two, or a week as in my case, or up to 6 weeks as in the case of my friend and several other patients I've worked with. The length of time the teeth are bound shut will depend on a number of factors including the way the patient heals and any issues during surgery.

These surgical hooks are also the reason traditional braces on the front surfaces of the teeth are required and things like lingual braces and Invisalign just aren't surgery-friendly.

Now let me introduce you to your new role as the Quarterback of your Jaw Surgery Team!

Notes: *Invisalign is a registered trademark with Align Technology, Inc. www.aligntech.com ; For more information regarding lingual braces, visit the American Lingual Orthodontic Association (ALOA) at www.lingualbraces.org*

You are the Quarterback & Team Captain

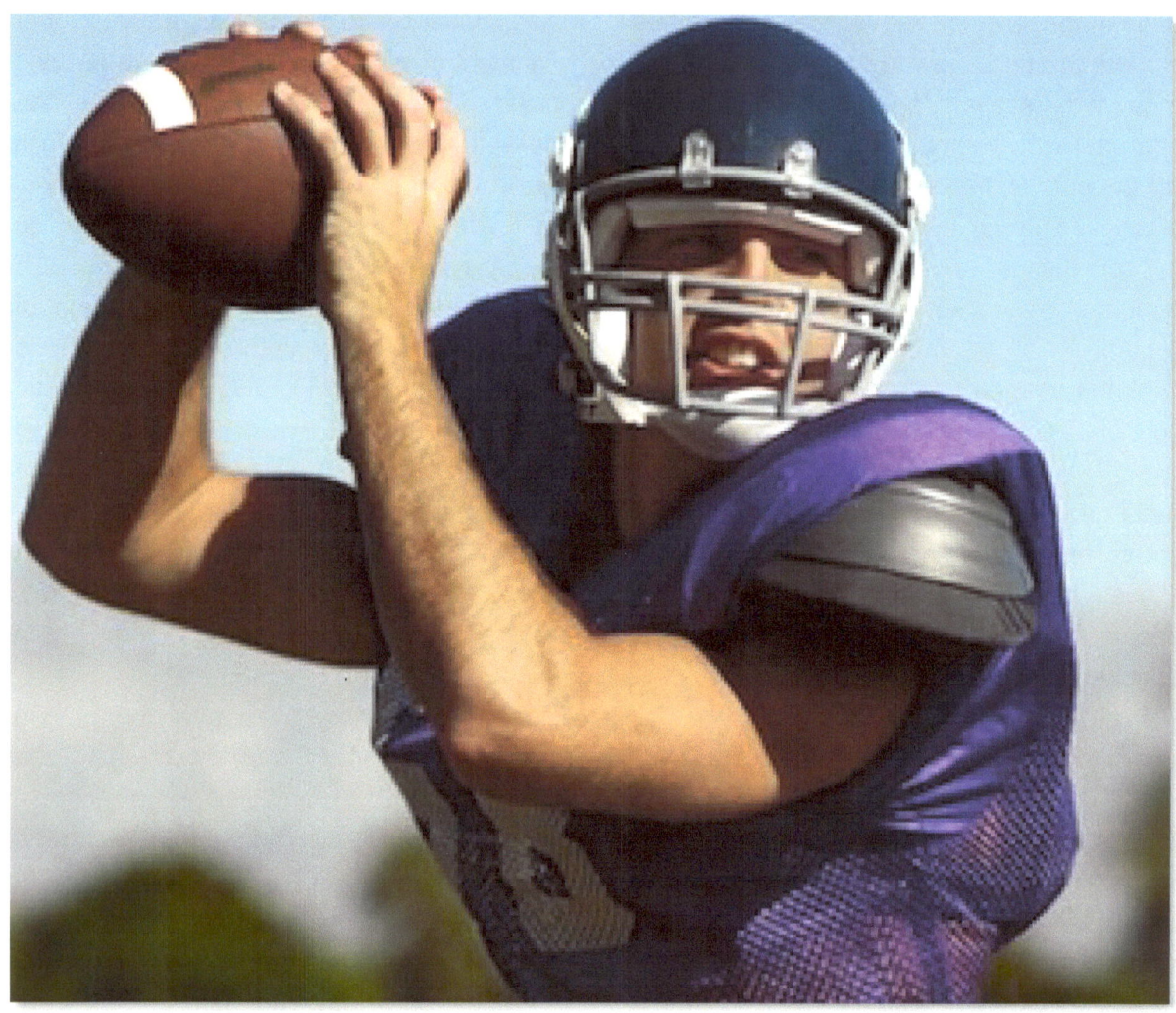

Your new role as Quarterback is to prepare yourself and your team for Game Day and Recovery. You will work with your Offensive Coordinators to ensure you have the answers to your questions, the information you need, prepare you for surgery and recovery, and to help you prepare your Defense for your surgery and recovery.

You will use the Playbook System to prepare your home, body and mind for surgery and recovery, including calculating your nutrition needs, menu planning, shopping lists, supplies, personal care and more. If you haven't already, please review the Training Camp section of the Jaw Recovery Playbook website for more in-depth information on what to expect and what you will experience throughout your surgery and recovery process.

Now -- Let's meet your TEAM!

As the Quarterback, your primary job before surgery is to meet with your Offensive Coordinators and to make sure all information is relayed to your Team. The Offensive Coordinators are any professionals involved in your treatment, including your General Dentist, Orthodontist, Surgeon and/or Surgical Team. Although most patients do not have a General Dentist actively involved in their orthodontics and surgical treatment, it is important to keep your dentist informed of your treatment with other professionals AND attend your annual or biannual cleanings to keep teeth and gums healthy.

A patient is referred to an orthodontist by their general dentist. The initial implication is that the patient has a malocclusion of some sort; a misalignment of the teeth. The orthodontist will perform an initial consultation and present the patient with options for treatment. Some patients have other complaints such as TMJ issues, breathing issues, speech issues, or tongue thrust. In most cases, this is when the patient learns he needs surgery, but we will discuss that further in a bit. The orthodontist will refer the patient to an oral & maxillofacial surgeon for another consultation and the two will coordinate the patient's care. Sometimes this coordination needs help from the patient to ensure both the orthodontist and the surgeon(s) stay on the same page.

Your TEAM is composed of any family or friends involved in your treatment and recovery. For many patients, the Team is a Mom and/or Dad, and possibly siblings or a spouse. Some patients have smaller Teams, and a few may have a Team of one: the patient, alone. Any Team composition is acceptable but it is beneficial to have at least one responsible adult prepared to assist during recovery, available to drive and pick-up the patient from surgery and available for the initial follow-up appointments.

As the patient, it is important to understand that the complete Jaw Surgery experience, from initial orthodontics referral to the surgery and recovery, then ultimately having the braces removed, can be overwhelming. It will not be overwhelming everyday but at times you will feel stressed and this can affect your mood, sleep, concentration, and make you feel irritable toward those around you. Managing stress throughout this treatment process will become significantly easier with the help of a well-informed Team. As non-patients, your Team cannot be expected to completely understand what you are feeling or going through -- don't leave them in the dark. This Offense Playbook will help you communicate effectively with all involved for your BEST chance at a FULL RECOVERY!

2

So I'm Having Jaw Surgery… Now What?

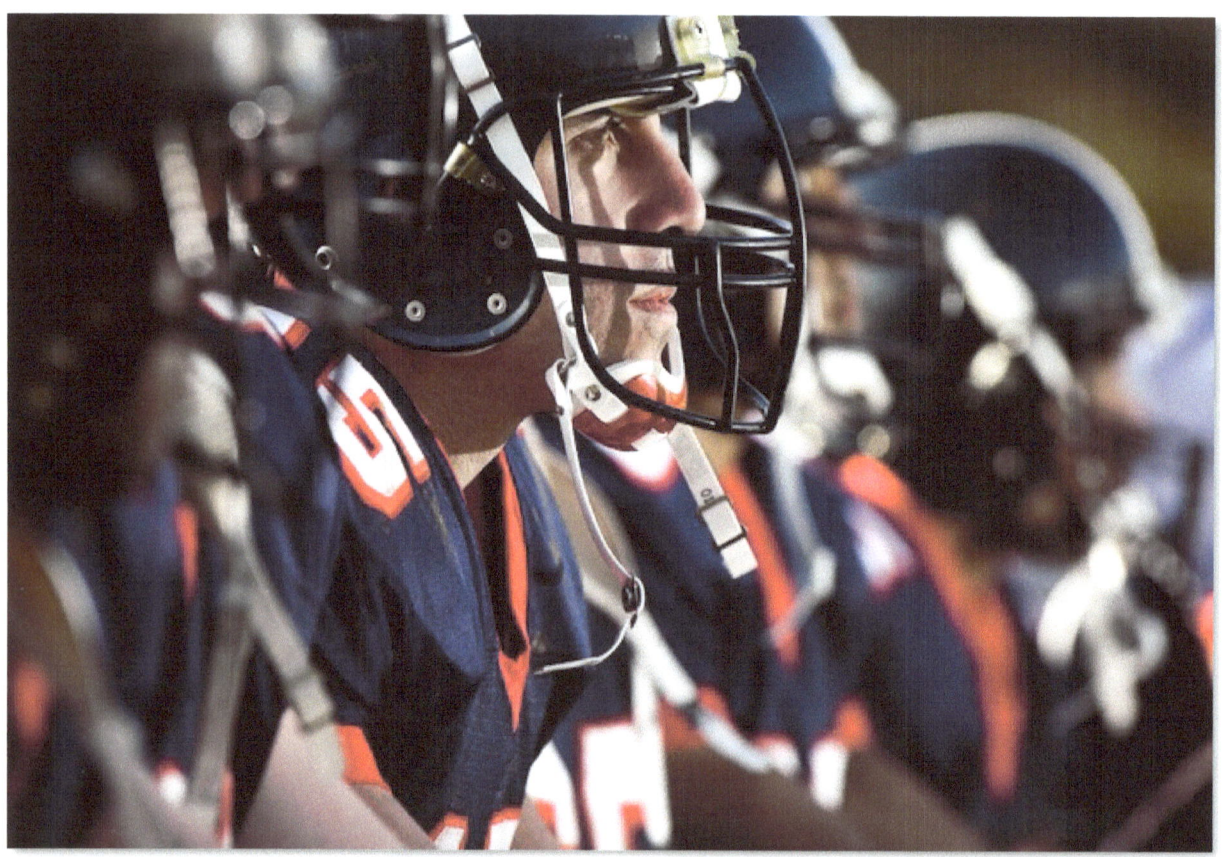

How Soon is "too soon" to Prepare?

As soon as you learn you will definitely need jaw surgery, many patients begin carousing the internet for information from other patients. We're naturally curious, as human beings, and this is normal…but it can also be extremely counterproductive. The majority of information available through internet searches consists of personal blogs and YouTube videos from other patients and this information is spotty at best. Patients generally do not provide detailed information regarding the important aspects of the surgery process, but instead focus on what all other patients focus on: pain, swelling, appearance, discomfort, and eating. This does not mean that such things are not important, but there are far more important factors patients should understand to better their chances of a complete or near-complete recovery. Even if some information is obtained, these personal blogs and videos tend to increase anxiety in patients and undermine communication efforts with surgeons and orthodontists.

You're welcome to search the internet for blogs and videos from past jaw surgery patients, but try to take all information with a grain of salt -- meaning, just because it was true for that person, does not make it true for you. Surgery procedures, policies, and experiences change from one patient to the next, and from one country or region to the next. Comparing can be interesting, but do not fall into the bad habit of assuming what was true for Patient A or Patient B will be true for you.

So if searching the internet is counterproductive, what should I do while I wait for surgery?

An excellent place to start your surgery preparations is with an appropriate outlook. When you meet your surgeon for your initial consult, he will often provide a tentative timeline for your treatment. In my case, the first surgeon suggested I would have braces for roughly 6-8 months and then I would undergo upper-jaw and lower-jaw procedures, after which I would complete my braces in approximately 3-4 months giving me a timeline of about a year, give or take a few months. Unfortunately, these timelines are nothing more than wild guesses -- educated guesses, but definitely arbitrary. The reality of the situation is that everyone's teeth move at a different pace and with differing degrees of efficacy. Some patients may not need braces to straighten teeth or close gaps, but are required to wear braces as part of surgery preparations.

When my braces went on for surgery preparation, I was aware that teeth move differently for every patient because I wore braces as a teenager. Although I did feel frustrated at times, I feel that my expectations for my surgery timeline were closer to realistic in that I did not believe I would be ready for surgery before the one-year mark. It actually took 16 months for me to reach surgery-ready - nearly double the predicted timeline.

Interestingly, when I made decisions for my orthodontics treatment I opted for self-ligating brackets, which are slightly smaller than traditional brackets and they contain a tiny latch that closes around the archwires. The self-ligating braces are said to cut treatment time in half, so if it took 16 months to reach surgery-ready with self-ligating braces, it likely would have taken over 2 years with traditional braces. That, to me, was worth the $1000.00 difference in the prices so I was happy I went with that option. This is something patients should consider, however, when making decisions regarding their surgery treatment but also when considering their timeline.

Care for your hardware -
Care for your teeth & gums!

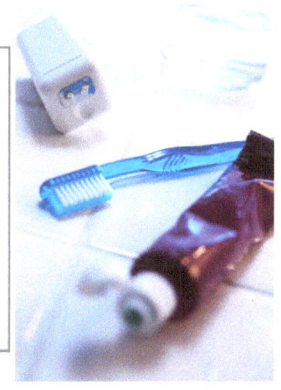

Proper oral hygiene will reduce risk of cavities and gum disease while you wear braces.

For those that have had braces in the past, this will seem a little monotonous, but CARE FOR YOUR TEETH, GUMS, & HARDWARE.

Make good use of a proxabrush to clean food and build-up from between brackets and take your time brushing to make certain the toothbrush makes contact with your teeth and gum-line to prevent irritation.

Flossing with braces is tricky, and you likely don't floss everyday in the first place, BUT do your best to at least floss a few times a week. Traditional floss is fine, but thicker floss will help clean between teeth better...and don't forget to RINSE. Use a good mouth rinse with fluoride to prevent cavities, especially since you can't effectively brush every part of your teeth and gums for the time being.

Whitening Teeth with Braces

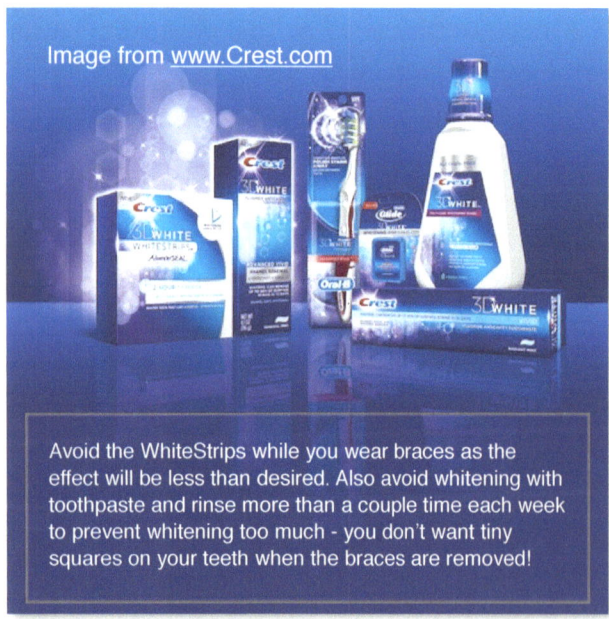

Avoid the WhiteStrips while you wear braces as the effect will be less than desired. Also avoid whitening with toothpaste and rinse more than a couple time each week to prevent whitening too much - you don't want tiny squares on your teeth when the braces are removed!

Twice a week, I would use my proxabrush with a whitening toothpaste to clean in-between each bracket, making sure to scrub the exposed surfaces of both teeth for several seconds before moving on to the next. Then I would brush with the whitening toothpaste using a standard toothbrush and rinse with a whitening rinse or standard fluoride rinse. As a grown-up, I drink coffee and tea, both of which stain teeth. I didn't want to bleach my teeth or whiten too much because the color would be too different once the brackets are removed -- but I wanted to lighten the staining a bit to keep my teeth presentable.

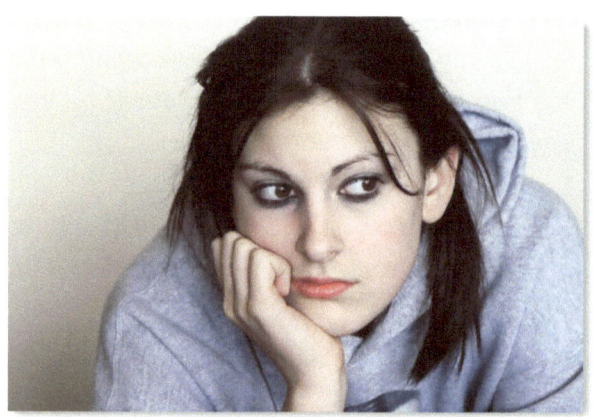

The road to surgery is usually a long one, so preparing in advance can seem like a waste of time. Many patients wait until they have an actual surgery date before they begin preparations, but there is a lot you can do now to better your chances of a successful surgery and full recovery.

Begin with an honest assessment of your health - including your current weight, fitness level, and nutrition. Do you currently exercise at least 4-5 days each week, for at least 30-45 minutes each day? Are you overweight? Underweight? Do you have any conditions that are affected by nutrition such as digestive issues or blood sugar issues (i.e. hypoglycemia, hyperglycemia, diabetes, acid-reflux)? Do you often have food cravings? Do you eat breakfast and at least two other meals each day? Do you know how many calories you consume on a regular basis? Or how much protein? Fiber? How much do you sleep and do you sleep on a regular schedule?

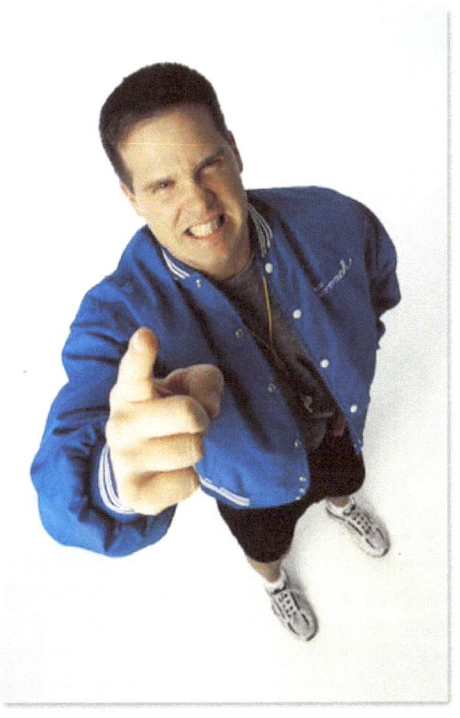

If you cannot confidently answer the sample list of health questions posed on the previous page, it's a safe bet that your next step should be adding a fitness plan and improving nutrition. I tell every patient that comes to me for help preparing for their jaw surgery: **"Recovery is approximately 30% attitude and 80% nutrition - if you aim for 110% recovery, even if you fall a little short you can still reach 100%."**

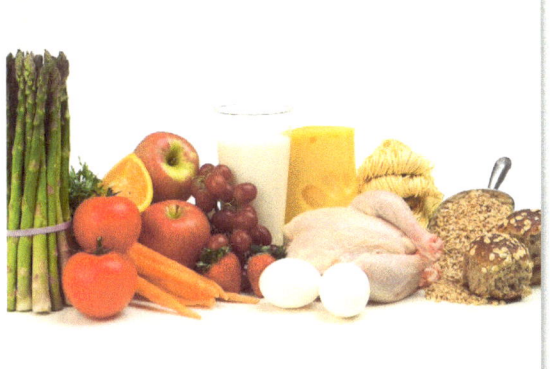

Proper nutrition, however, will vary from one patient to the next. I engage in rigorous activity for at least 45-60 minutes several days each week and also lift weights for healthy muscle, which helps maintain healthy body weight by keeping metabolism strong. For my nutrition, I usually consume at least 1500 to 1800 calories with close to 100 grams of protein each day and at least 25 grams of fiber. This may be too much for some other female patients, or too little for male patients. It may also be too little for a female patient who does more than me with regard to weight-training and cardiovascular workouts. In the nutrition section, I provide a very basic system for determining what YOU need now, to help improve your nutrition while you prepare for surgery.

This will help make your recovery nutrition a lot easier!

If you currently engage in zero exercise beyond your everyday tasks, it's strongly recommended that you begin as soon as possible. The healthier your body is the faster it will heal and the more efficiently it will heal, meaning you stand a greater chance of a FULL recovery. Patients in their teens are much more flexible with such things, but any patient over 18-years-old should be monitoring their nutrition and exercising regularly to give their body the best fighting chance.

Sufficient hydration is key for healthy cell function throughout the body. Every part of your body requires water to function, and if you do not drink enough water, your body has to either take fluids from itself or start operating at a level below optimal. In either case, you will not be able to recover easily from major jaw surgery unless you improve your hydration so it's best to start now.

Most experts suggest 8 cups of water per day, which is 64oz. This is only sufficient if you do absolutely nothing all day. If you are active with regular exercise, you should drink considerably more water. I consume over 100oz each day - which I measure by refilling a 20oz cup. When water is boring I add Stevia (which doesn't affect blood sugar) and True Lime crystalized lime juice (www.truecitrus.com). Avoid sports drinks (such as Gatorade) and diet drinks (including vitamin waters), and avoid high-sodium foods for best water absorption.

> The recommended 64oz. of water each day is a minimum. If you do nothing but stay in bed all day, 64oz. may suffice, but if you exercise you should consume significantly more.

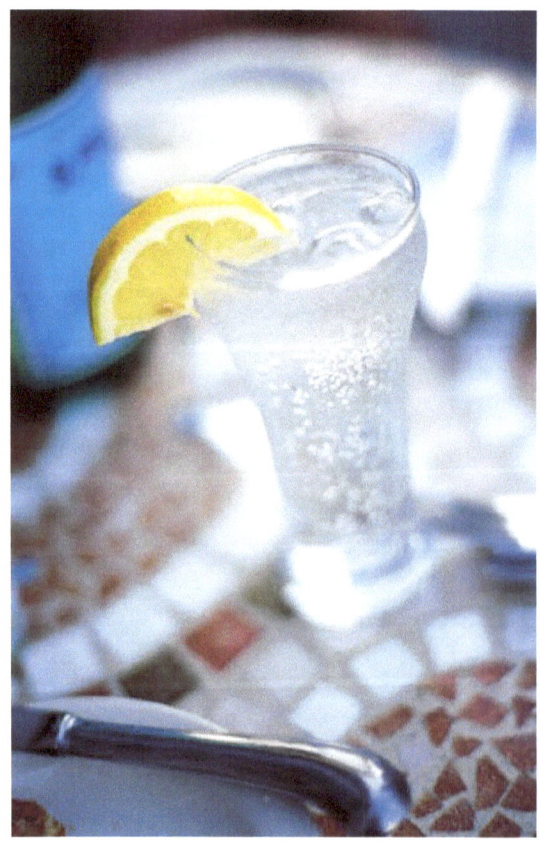

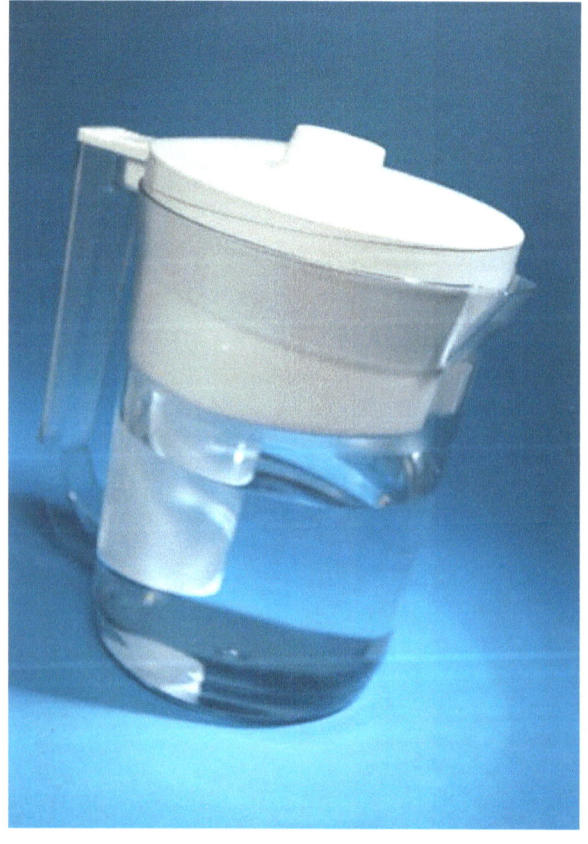

Manage Your Own Treatment

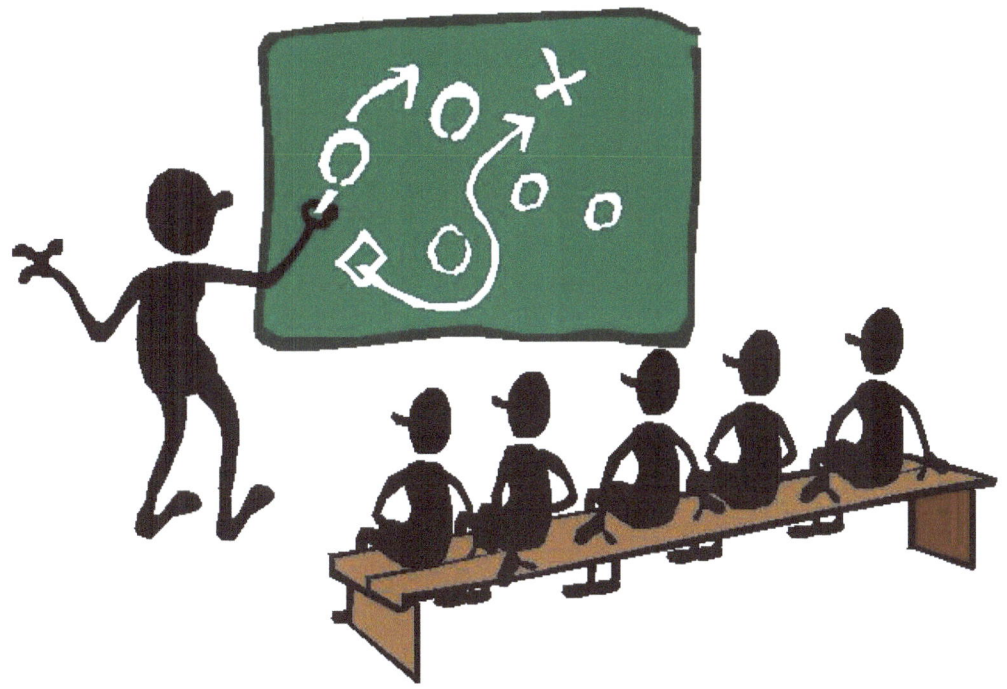

A major part of preparing for Jaw Surgery is the management of your treatment in the meantime. That treatment includes attending your General Dentist appointments for cleanings and check-ups which are usually once every 6 months or once a year, depending on insurance coverage. This preventative treatment is essential for the health of your teeth and gums. It would be a shame to go through the process of braces and surgery only to have your teeth full of cavities or in need of extraction!

Making and keeping your appointments with your orthodontist is also extremely important. **After all, the longer it takes to prepare for surgery the longer you have to wait for surgery.** Keeping your appointments for orthodontic adjustments and check-ups will help keep you on track, and get you to surgery sooner.

You will not have many appointments with your surgeon. After the initial consult, you will likely not see your surgeon again until your orthodontist says she thinks you are ready for surgery. Then you will see the surgeon for a visit similar to your initial consult (meaning - be prepared for a LONG visit almost every time). Once the surgeon completes the assessment, he will consult with your orthodontist regarding continued adjustments needed to prepare you for surgery, or he will discuss with you a plan to set up a surgery date.

It is important to note, however, that until you are given a set date for surgery, you should refrain from assuming you are ready for surgery. You will be surgery-ready when the surgeon feels your teeth are in the best possible places for the best possible results - and not a moment sooner. I went to my surgeon three times and each time my orthodontist felt I was ready, based on the surgeon's previous instructions. Each time I was sent back to my orthodontist for more adjustments. Try to understand that this is going to be frustrating but it's necessary to improve your chances of success. You do not want a surgeon to rush your procedures only to botch the work and leave you in need of multiple surgeries to repair your jaw or face - right? Try to remain patient…

Improve your orthodontic treatment and treatment speed by talking with your orthodontist and taking control of your treatment. As mentioned, I opted for self-ligating braces which my orthodontist explained would cut my treatment time in half (approximately). It took 16 months to get to surgery from the time my braces were put on, though, and I was initially told to expect surgery in 6-8 months. When I would have an appointment with my orthodontist, if I wasn't clear on what changes he was making and what changes I should expect to see in my teeth, I would ask him to tell me what he was doing and why. This allowed me to know what to expect when watching my teeth move between that appointment and my next.

Now, granted, you can't really watch your teeth moving, but every day I would check my bite and teeth while brushing, flossing, putting on makeup, or washing up. If I noticed that the teeth were moving more than I thought they would, or if it had been a week and the teeth hadn't moved at all, I would call my orthodontist and go back early. With the self-ligating braces I was in for appointments almost every 3-4 weeks because he could adjust them at a faster pace. I would also go back, sometimes without an appointment, if I was in the neighborhood and needed a wire clipped or wanted them to check something. By taking this proactive approach to my treatment, I am certain I sped up the process to get to surgery. Considering it took more than twice what I expected to get to surgery-ready, I imagine if I had waited for each scheduled appointment and not been as proactive with my treatment, it might have been 2-3 years before I was ready for surgery. This is important to remember.

Optimize Time Spent with Your Surgeon

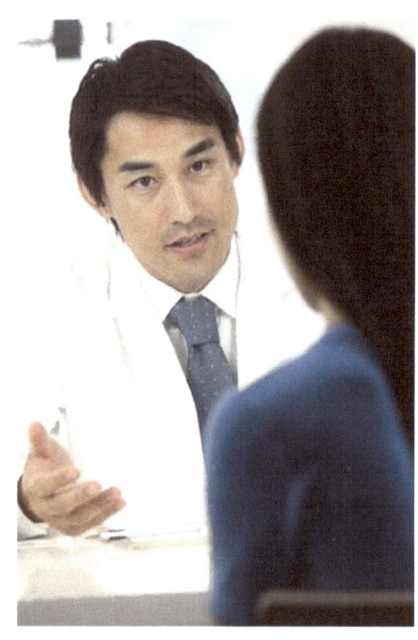

You will find that after leaving almost every appointment with your surgeon you will have forgotten to ask something or he will have said something you forgot or didn't completely understand. **Don't worry - we all do this!**

There are ways, however, to get the most out of each appointment. Start with a notebook. Make it a clean, new notebook dedicated specifically to your appointments with your providers (e.g. orthodontist, surgeon, etc.). As soon as you have a scheduled appointment, write the date and time at the top of a clean page in the notebook. Now, every time you have a question about something regarding your surgery, treatment, or anything related, write it down! Then bring the notebook with you to every appointment.

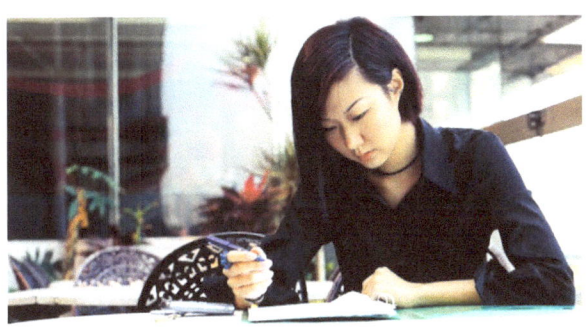

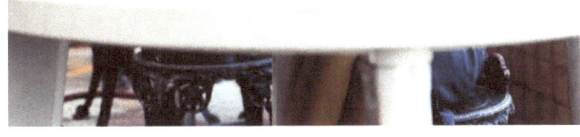

Take notes during your appointments. In between appointments, write down questions or concerns you have so you are sure to remember to discuss them at your next visit.

You can do this on your phone with most smartphones too, if that's easier. I found the notebook was more effective because I remember things better when I've manually written them down. I also found it was faster to jot down notes by hand during my appointments when I would get answers to my questions or if the surgeon would say something I felt I should remember.

Your surgeon is NOT a mind-reader, and in most cases your surgeon has never been a jaw surgery patient. This means, he will never truly understand what you are feeling, and he will never be able to guess every possible question or concern you have. **If you don't ask, you will never know for certain!**

Your questions will help your surgeon also! Be CLEAR when asking questions - if you think your surgeon doesn't understand, explain again. If there's something YOU don't understand, ask him to explain. By asking questions, you give your surgeon a better idea of what his patients are experiencing which he can then apply to his interactions with other patients.

Many patients don't ask their surgeons questions when they should and instead they continue to wonder and worry. This is counterproductive because it increases anxiety about the surgery when the patient might otherwise be able to relax. It also undermines your ability to feel confidence with your surgeon, his team, your orthodontist, and anyone else involved.

Instead of stressing and wondering about the little things you're curious or concerned about, talk with your surgeon and orthodontist for answers and information. Recovery after surgery is much MUCH easier when you're mind is clear and your mood is positive!

I strongly urge patients under 18-years-old to discuss their concerns, questions and fears with a parent, guardian, sibling, or other caregiver for support.

Manage Your Own Treatment - RECAP:

1. **Get a notebook for your orthodontic and surgery treatment process.** This notebook is for orthodontic and surgery appointments ONLY. If you have a two-subject notebook, you can separate one half for orthodontic notes and the other half for surgery notes. If you have a three-subject notebook you can use the third section for notes from the Jaw Recovery Playbook System to help guide your own recovery planning.

2. **Each time you have a new appointment scheduled with your orthodontist, write the date and time at the top of a clean page in that section.** Every time you have an appointment scheduled with your surgeon, write the date and time at the top of a clean page in that section.

3. **Underneath the scheduled appointment title on the page, write any questions, notes, concerns, or observations you have that come to mind in the time between appointments.** Leave room to write answers while you are at the appointment so you can take notes fast to keep appointments efficient.

4. **When the orthodontist or surgeon speaks at your appointment, have your notebook ready to jot down notes.** This will be crucial when going between providers because you want to make sure that YOU understand what is going on so if you think the surgeon wasn't clear with your orthodontist (when they spoke) you have notes to help encourage the orthodontist to double-check or get clarification from the surgeon, and vice versa.

5. **It doesn't matter if you are under 18-years-old** and your parents attend every appointment with you, **if you are not taking the initiative and working to manage your own appointments and treatment, you will feel helpless and lost.** Be the Quarterback. Be the Team Captain. Guide your own treatment and encourage good, clear, and consistent communication between all people involved.

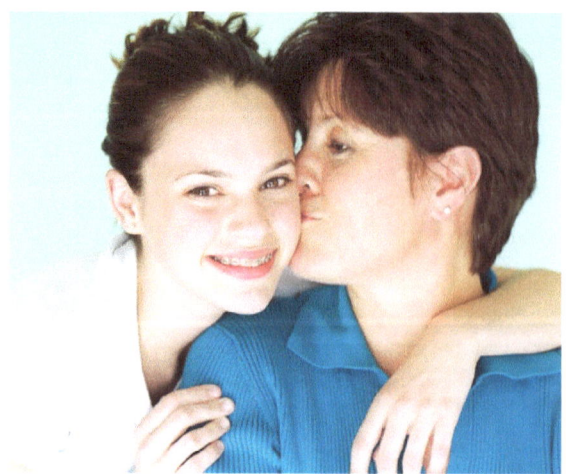

YOU are responsible for YOU –
The more you do for yourself,
the easier your treatment and

3
Skincare Before & After Surgery

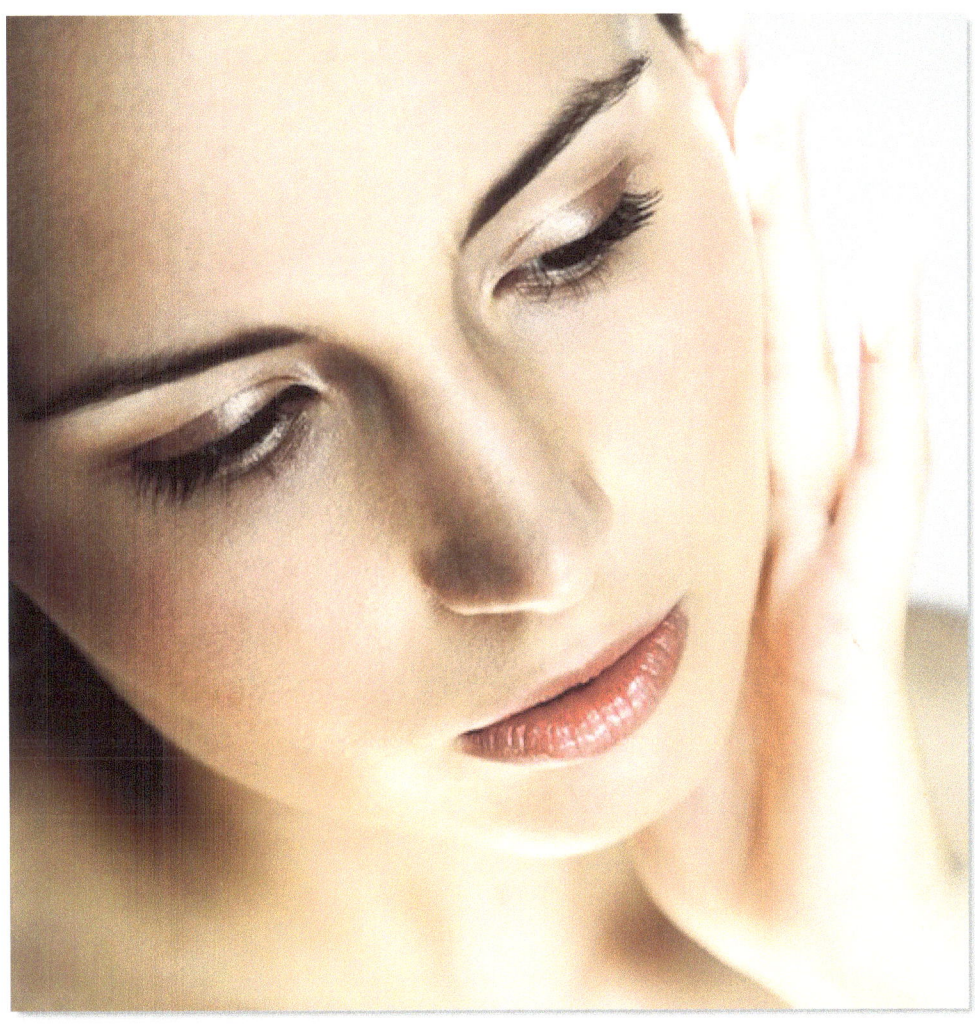

Skincare is particularly important after jaw surgery, for both male and female patients, but caring for your skin becomes easier if you start to develop good habits long before surgery. Younger patients may not realize the amount of stress placed on their skin and lips from surgery and recovery, and older patients may overlook the implications. Skincare will enable your skin to maintain elasticity so the swelling and exposure during recovery do not cause any permanent issues such as sagging or wrinkles. This is true for younger patients and older patients alike.

Washing with Care

Avoid using a standard bar soap on your face. This is particularly targeting male patients but all patients, men and women, should use a face-specific cleanser. Facial cleansers are designed to clean off makeup, skin oils, and any gunk collected from sweat and exposure throughout the day. For those with problem skin, including acne and dryness, a facial cleanser is ideal because it will reduce irritation which is a common factor for acne-prone skin types, and the facial cleanser will also prevent over-drying while helping the skin on your face balance for a more even tone and texture.

Gentle cleansers are available in almost every grocery store and drug store. Brands like Neutrogena (www.neutrogena.com) offer affordable face wash options that are widely available, with skin-type specific varieties such as "for combination skin" or "for sensitive skin." I use BareMinerals makeup and skincare products so that's what I continued using throughout my recovery (www.bareescentuals.com).

It's best to wash your face separate from your typical shower washing. That way you can put more focus on cleaning properly and prevent over-drying your face since many people use hotter water in the shower.

When washing your face, apply a small amount of warm water to your face and hands. Rub your hands together with a small amount of facial cleanser in them to warm the cleanser and lather it a bit then apply to your face using your fingertips to massage in gentle circles. This helps really clean away dirt and oils, and work the cleanser into pores. Rinse with warm water then pat dry with a towel.

Avoid using hot water (steaming) on your face as this will over-dry your skin.

After surgery, your face may have some feeling in it right away, or it may feel completely numb. There may be tingling but the numbness may simply be a lack of any sensation. This can be dangerous if you use hot water because you may unknowingly burn your skin if your hands can tolerate warmer temperatures than your face. It's best to grow accustomed to using warm water instead of steaming hot water when washing your face so you're prepared for after surgery.

Toner and Astringent

Acne-prone skin can benefit from a toner or astringent. These salicylic acid-based liquids can sting when applied to acne, open-blemishes, or to irritated skin, so take care when using for the first time.

Toner is a similar liquid that can sting if applied to irritated skin but generally has a gentle feel and helps reduce pores by cleaning out dirt and oils. This can also leave skin feeling and looking refreshed and help reduce the effects of aging.

After washing with a facial cleanser and warm (not hot) water, pat your face dry and apply enough toner or astringent to a cotton pad or cotton ball to soak through. Gently rub the cotton with toner or astringent on face, across your forehead, over your nose including the creases at the sides of most noses, on cheeks and chin. Avoid skin near your eyes. Let the liquid dry before applying moisturizer.

If you regularly use makeup, using a toner can reduce the appearance of pores and uneven skin tone, depending on the quality and ingredients.

For men, using a toner will help reduce the size and appearance of pores which generally fill with oils and dirt. Breakouts associated with shaving will reduce with regular use of toner or astringent as well.

Moisturize to Protect and Prevent

A quality facial moisturizer is one of the most important things you can apply to your skin. Moisturizing prevents dryness and reduces the development of wrinkles and fine lines by keeping the skin soft and flexible.

Moisturizing your face is not just for women. There are now plenty of product lines designed specifically for men, with masculine fragrances and shaving-safe ingredients. After shaving, men can apply a light moisturizer using a fingertip massage similar to when you wash up. If you spend a lot of time outdoors, use a moisturizer with SPF in it for protection from the sun when you moisturize in the morning. At night, feel free to use a heavier moisturizer such as anti-aging creams for deeper moisture penetration.

For women, moisturizers with SPF are great for daytime. Regardless of age, an anti-aging moisturizer applied at night as part of a skincare regimen will keep skin moist, flexible, and young for much longer than untreated skin.

Eye-safe moisturizers are available in different types. Some offer deep moisturizing for healthy-looking skin around the eyes while others offer plumping to reduce the appearance of crows' feet or wrinkles. Tinted under-eye moisturizers help reduce dark circles -- but you can reduce dark circles the old fashioned way by getting enough sleep and drinking sufficient water.

Shaving Products (Men)

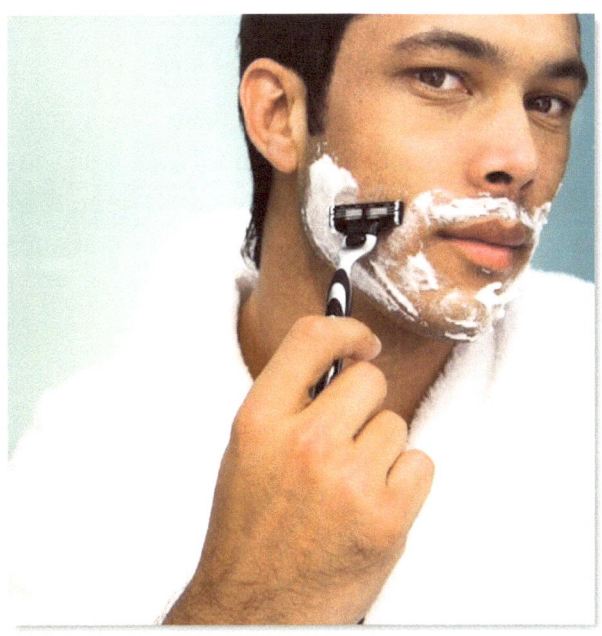

Quality shaving products will help maintain your skin's elasticity which will reduce visible aging and help your skin recovery faster and easier after surgery. Opt for a shaving gel instead of foam; the gel still foams but stays thicker for better protection from the blades of your razor. Avoid cheap disposable razors. Although the cost is significantly greater, a better quality razor will reduce skin damage and irritation while cutting the thick facial hair closer and more precisely. This will reduce nicks and cuts in conjunction with the quality shaving gel and help your skin appear cleaner, softer, and well cared-for.

Makeup Products (Women)

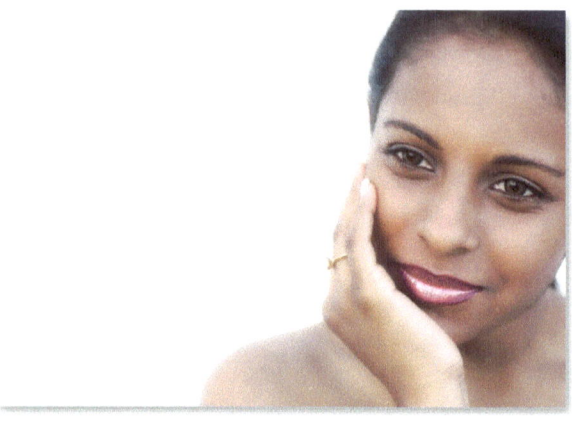

In general, the better the quality, the better the makeup products will be for your skin. As I mentioned, I favor BareMinerals products but there are plenty of quality makeup options within any budget range.

Never sleep in your makeup. This leads to problems with skin, including acne. It will also settle in early wrinkles making them appear deeper and more noticeable. Eye makeup left on overnight can also irritate your eyes and lead to eye infections or conjunctivitis - Not very attractive!

Likewise, never apply makeup to dirty skin. You will only be rubbing dirt and oils into your pores making them appear darker. You will also be rubbing makeup into fine lines and wrinkles making them more visible.

What About Exfoliating?

Exfoliating is entirely up to you. For those unfamiliar with the concept, exfoliating facial cleansers generally contain some form of sand-like scrubbing substance to help scrub away dead skin cells on the surface of your face. This helps maintain a more youthful, healthy appearance and also helps improve the absorption of toner, astringent, moisturizer, and other treatments. Think of it like treating wood or painting a wall. You sand the wall first or sand down the wood furniture first then clean off the surface before painting or applying stain. This helps even the tone and texture of the wall or furniture. Using an exfoliating scrub on your face works in a similar fashion for other products.

Exfoliating too much can leave skin irritated so if you choose to exfoliate, using an apricot scrub or other facial scrub, it's best to use it only a few times a week to prevent irritation.

Hand Care

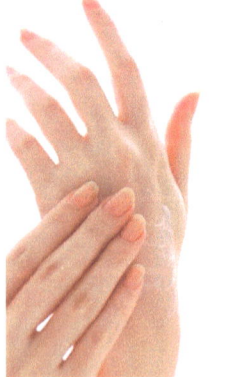

After surgery, one thing I noticed was almost chronic dry skin on my hands. I assumed it was from the tape from the IVs, which I had on both hands during surgery. It took several weeks before I found a lotion that helped - an intensive dry skin hand cream from A v e e n o (www.aveeno.com).

Lip Care

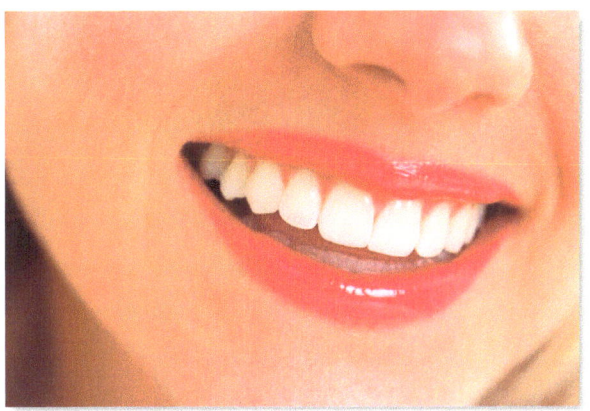

You can exfoliate your lips to prevent or reduce dryness and chapping. A simple homemade lip scrub, easy to make and apply, can dramatically improve the appearance and feel of your lips which will help during your recovery but also help prevent frequent-chapping commonly associated with braces.

Warm equal parts honey and olive (or coconut) oil in a small cup or bowl. A teaspoon of each is sufficient. You want to warm the mix for 5 seconds in the microwave, enough for the honey to stir easily but not burn you. Stir in a teaspoon of granular sugar. This has to be regular sugar and not a sugar substitute. With your fingers, gently rub the sugar mix into your upper and lower lips, using small circular motions and side-to-side gentle scrubbing motions. Wet a cloth with warm water and squeeze out, then use the cloth to wipe off your lips. Apply a lip balm or treatment such as Blistex Medicated Lip Ointment (www.blistex.com) or other lip balms and moisturizers.

Hair Care

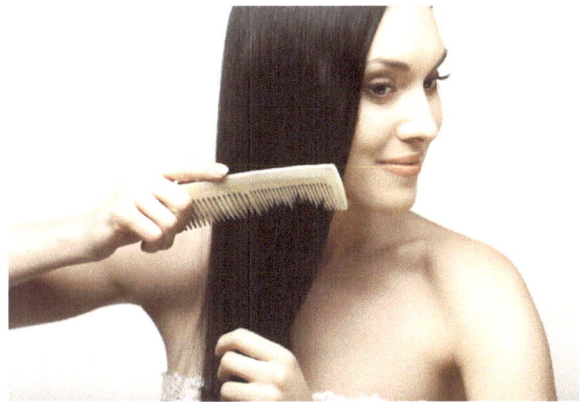

Although not necessarily "skin care" it's helpful to develop a regimen with your hair care that you will be able to manage after surgery. I anticipated my facial swelling to be worse than it was - I thought I would struggle too much holding a hairdryer and flat iron so I decided to get a short, almost pixie-like cut. It wasn't necessary, but I liked it.

You will want a haircut that you can manage (and tolerate!) with very little effort.

> A low-maintenance haircut will help you feel better after surgery because you will be able to wash and lightly style with minimal effort. It makes a difference!

4
Basic Nutrition

"About 80% of your Jaw Surgery success will depend on YOUR nutrition and health before and after surgery." ~ Sasha

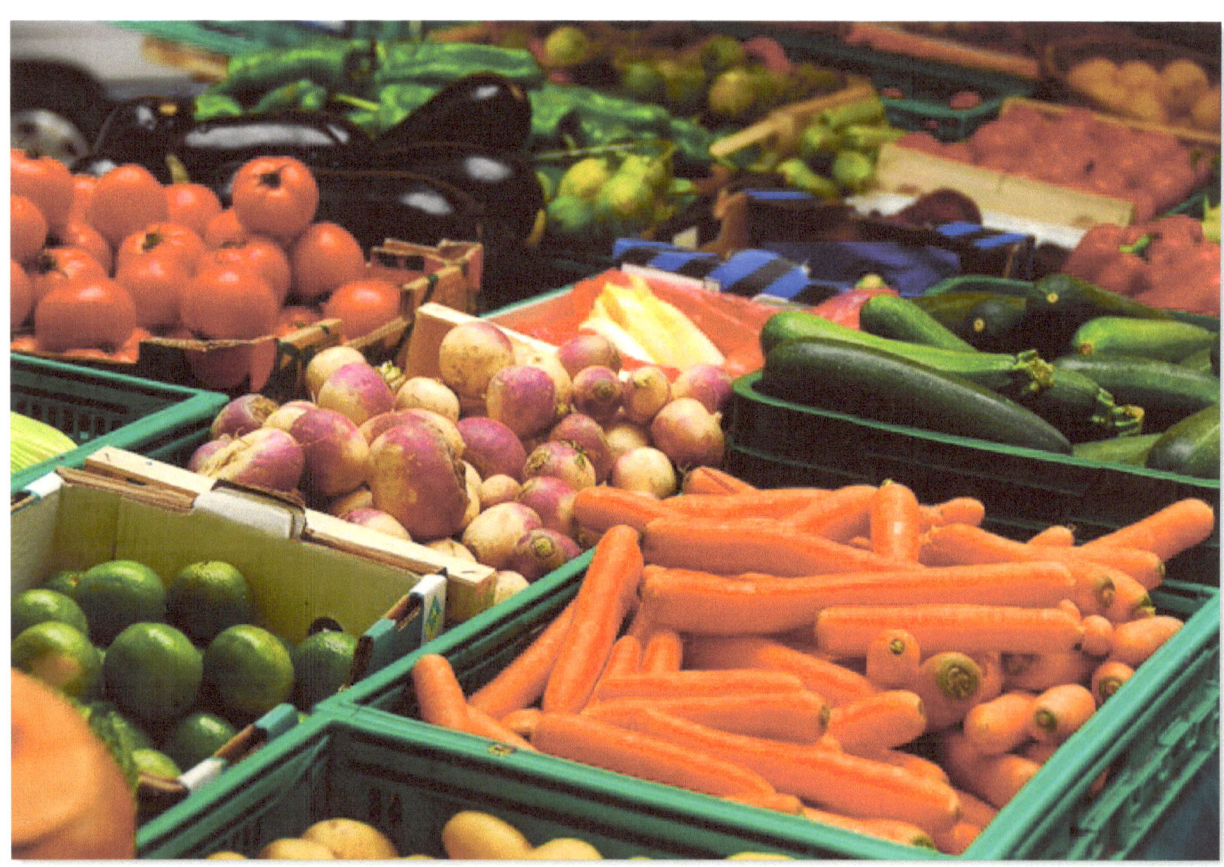

Macronutrients

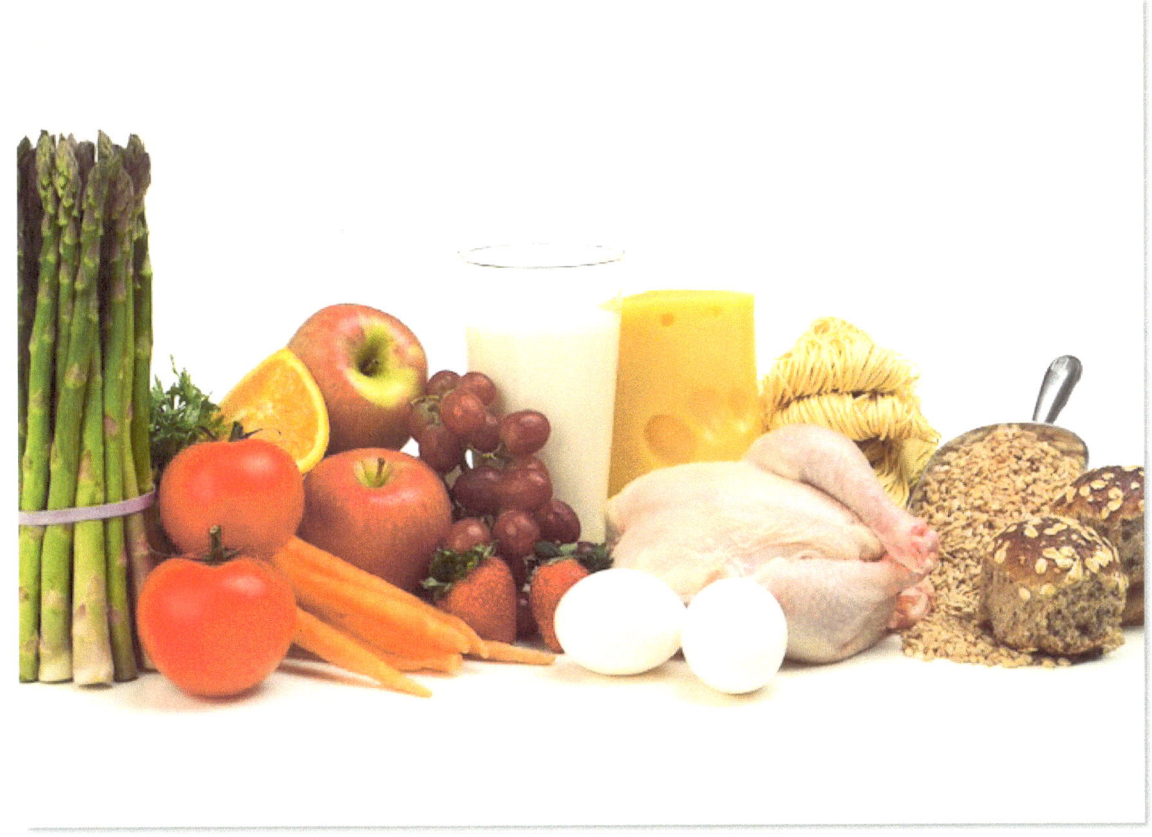

At the very basic level, macronutrients are nutrients the body needs in large quantities in order to function properly and maintain health. Protein is a macronutrient, as are carbohydrates and lipids (fats). These are measured in grams, as opposed to milligram and microgram measurements found on vitamin and supplement labels.

Protein provides essential tools for your body to manage muscle and connective-tissue health, and any excess protein consumed, beyond the protein needed by your body for the basic functions, is converted into energy. **Carbohydrates** fuel your body's cells, providing energy for basic functions as well as energy to support your daily activities. If you consume too few carbs, your body has to take protein and fat from your body and diet to produce sufficient energy, which is the basis for low-carb diets but not necessarily the most efficient method of managing your health. If you consume too many carbs, however, the excess is typically converted and stored for later use which is often a factor in weight-gain.

Lipids are fats and comprise the most abundant source of stored fuel within the body. Lipids are also a component of the membranes surrounding cells and some hormones are lipid-hormones, such as estrogen. These hormones help regulate bodily functions - in the case of estrogen, the lipid-hormone helps regulate the female reproductive cycle. Protein is also involved in regulation, in particular the regulation of body fat.

Water is considered a macronutrient because the body requires it to survive and the body requires significant amounts of water to maintain health and internal function. Water regulates the body's temperature, which you may recall from grade school health class - when we sweat, the lost fluids cool our bodies to help keep us from overheating.

Many people, especially women, will notice their bodies hold more water (water retention) around the time of their monthly cycle but the body can also look or feel "puffy" if too little water is consumed (or if you consume too much sodium).

Drinking too little water each day can affect bathroom trips as well, in the form of constipation, especially if sufficient fiber is consumed but not enough water to manage it. Urine will also appear darker and in smaller quantities as the body dehydrates, and a consistently insufficient amount of water each day can promote urinary tract issues including infections.

Recommended Daily Nutrition

To maintain a generally safe level of health, it is recommended that roughly 45-65% of your daily calories come from carbohydrates. **Carbohydrates are 4 calories per 1 gram, so if you consume 2000 calories a day and 50% of those calories are from carbohydrates that is about 1000 calories or 250 grams of carbs.** A standard 2oz serving of pasta, for example, provides about 40 grams of carbohydrates which would then be about 16% of your carbs for the day. This doesn't seem too bad, but the trick to maintaining weight with balanced carbohydrates is to avoid consuming too many carbs at one time -- excess beyond what your body can use will increase bodyweight over time.

Approximately 10-35% of your daily calories should come from protein, as recommended by the National Institutes of Health. In a 2000 calorie diet, 22% is about 440 calories. **One gram of protein provides 4 calories, like carbohydrates, so this would be 110 grams of protein.** This seems like a LOT to most people, unless you are a bodybuilder or diligently monitoring your own nutrition. I mentioned earlier that I consume an average of 100+ grams of protein per day, usually with 25-35 grams protein per meal, eating three meals a day, plus additional protein in my snacks.

Despite years of contradictory advice from the diet realm, **lipids are essential for health and we are given the recommendation of 20-35% of our daily calories coming from fats.** These fats are very easy to consume in the form of olive oil, grapeseed oil, coconut oil, and also supplements such as fish oil. **Twenty percent of 2000 calories is 400 calories; lipids provide 9 calories per gram so 400 calories is approximately 44 grams.** A tablespoon of grapeseed oil drizzled over a salad adds 120 calories which is over 1/4 the daily goal if on a 2000 calorie diet.

It is important to remember, however, that these RDAs, or Recommended Daily Allowances, are really only a blanket-guideline meant to be adjusted for each individual based on the different needs of that individual. These values are a good place to start, but individual factors should be considered before adhering to the RDAs listed here as if they were standard.

Individual Diet Factors

1. Is your current bodyweight healthy, overweight, obese, or underweight?

2. Do you sleep on a regular schedule, getting between 6 and 8 hours of sleep each night? Do you oversleep? Do you take naps?

3. Do you eat on a regular schedule? How often do you have cravings? How often do you skip meals?

4. Do you workout on a regular schedule, engaging in at least 30-45 minutes of activity at least 3 days a week? Do you do any weight-training to maintain healthy muscle?

5. Do you drink more than 64oz of water each day? When not drinking water, do you consume soda, diet beverages of any type, sports drinks, or energy drinks?

6. Are your moods relatively stable or do you tend to feel down, bored, sad, or depressed? If you experience these "blah" feelings, how often do they affect you?

7. How well do you manage stress? A better question may be to consider how often you feel stressed out?

8. Do you experience any heightened anxiety (separate from the anxiety associated with the anticipation of jaw surgery)?

9. Do you cook for yourself or live with someone who does the cooking? How often do you eat out and when you do, what type of foods do you eat while out?

10. How would you rate your overall energy levels? Do you feel like you have the energy to perform well at work or school throughout the day? Do you feel exhausted during the day?

These considerations are things that are affected by and influence your overall health. If you exercise on a regular basis, at least 3 days per week, and you eat on a schedule with sufficient nutrients and water, you will find that other aspects of your health seem to improve including your sleep patterns, your food cravings, your moods and stress management. You will also find it gets easier to maintain a healthy lifestyle once you implement small changes and make them habitual.

The information here can help you organize your efforts to improve your health and fitness before surgery which will set your body up for the absolute BEST chance of successful healing after surgery. **The sooner you start working on small health and fitness changes, the easier things will become.** In addition, the longer you work on your health and fitness before surgery, the better! **Jumping into a workout routine a month before your procedure isn't going to be as effective at improving your health as starting a regular exercise routine 12 months in advance.**

Regardless of your activity levels, you will need to avoid active exercise during the initial 6 weeks after surgery and many patients will have to wait up to 4 months post-surgery before they can engage in regular exercise again. This is due to post-surgery anemia, from the blood loss during surgery.

In my case, I was not aware of the anemia until I tried to go back to exercising about 5 weeks after surgery. After pushing myself through two workouts in week 5, I began experiencing terrible anemia symptoms and it took 4 months to recovery from that point. I discuss anemia in greater detail in the Game Day and Recovery Playbook.

~ ~ ~ ~ ~ ~ ~ ~ ~ ~

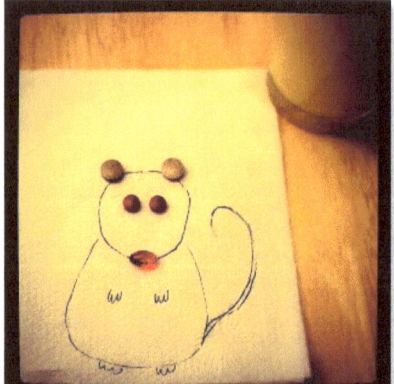

This is 'Ferrous' Bueller.

A mouse of the *mus ferrous* variety, or Iron Mouse.

The ears and eyes are two different types of iron in supplement-form, and the nose is Docusate to counteract the negative side-effects of too much iron. The glass in the upper-right corner contains Recovery Formula which has sufficient Vitamin C to aid iron absorption.

This was my nightly regimen for four months as I recovered slowly from severe anemia symptoms. Symptoms I might never have felt if I hadn't pushed myself to workout in week 5, so soon after surgery. I don't mention it to scare you, just to make a point.

It's worth taking the extra time to heal!

Micronutrients

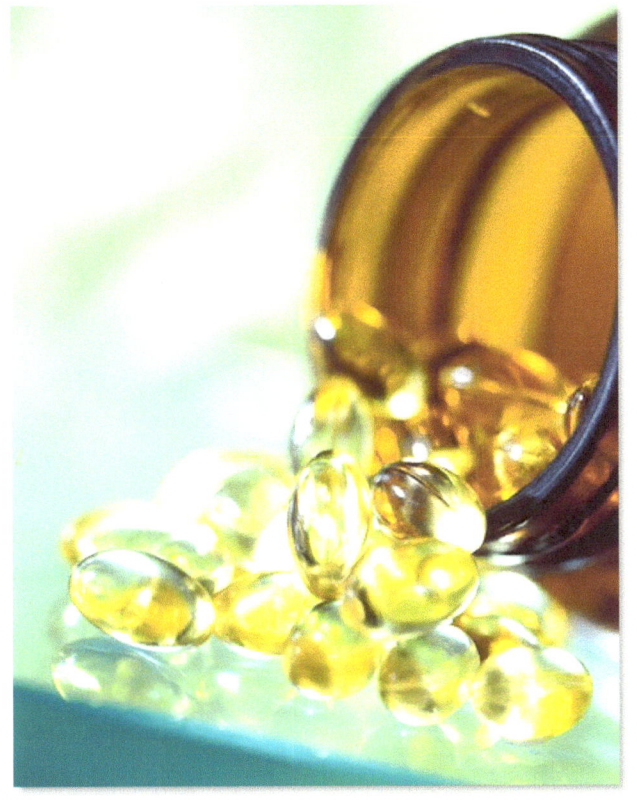

In contrast to macronutrients, the micronutrients are nutrients needed in small amounts by the body. Generally, micronutrients are vitamins and minerals. While macronutrients are measured in grams, denoting larger quantities, the micronutrients are measured in milligrams (mg) and micrograms (mcg).

Most micronutrients are water-soluble, which means you can consume large quantities safely even though you only need a small amount. For example, B vitamins are beneficial for nervous system health, metabolism, and a variety of other bodily functions. We can absorb our B vitamins from foods but many people supplement with tablets. Vitamin B12 is needed in a very small amount by the body - adults have an RDA of 1.8 mcg - but supplements provide large amounts of B12, usually 500mcg, 1000mcg, or more. Interestingly, the body stores enough vitamin B12 to sustain function for years even if you consume no additional vitamin B12.

A few micronutrients are fat-soluble, however, and these vitamins can be toxic if consumed in too large a dose. **The fat-soluble vitamins are Vitamin A, Vitamin D, Vitamin E, and Vitamin K.** Most people do not need supplements for any of these fat-soluble vitamins, with the exception of Vitamin D which some people take under the guidance of their physician. **Unless your general physician directs you to take Vitamin A, D, E, or K, it is best to avoid them as far as supplements go. You get plenty from food.**

During my recovery from jaw surgery, I added Vitamin B12 along with a B-Complex supplement containing Folic Acid to aid absorption. This was for general health due to the change in diet but primarily I wanted to provide my body with sufficient B vitamins to support nervous system operations. A major aspect of jaw surgery is the risk of nerve damage in the face. The nerves are generally not cut but they are exposed and moved around, stretched and irritated causing them to shut down temporarily. Sort of like if you touch a caterpillar and it curls up defensively but then over time it will uncurl and go about its business. Your nerves don't curl up but they do "turn off" in a sense which removes all (or almost all) sensation until they begin to recover. The recovery feels like tingling or "pins & needles" and some patients confuse this sensation with pain.

I also consumed an iron supplement, after learning how bad my post-surgery anemia was. Iron is a tricky supplement, in my opinion. If you consume iron with something high in calcium, the calcium blocks your ability to absorb and maximize the iron. For best absorption, you should consume the iron supplement with something high in Vitamin C - which aids absorption. That being said, many juices are fortified with calcium so you can't simply drink a glass of juice with the iron supplements without checking the calcium content.

Iron also has an unpleasant side-effect. The typical iron supplement is composed of ferrous sulfate which is not the most effective form of iron so much of the ferrous sulfate is not absorbed and instead it passes through the body and causes constipation. For this reason, when a doctor prescribes iron supplements, he also often prescribes a gentle stool softener (not a laxative). If you take the stool softener, be sure to consume an additional glass or two of water to prevent dehydration.

Calculate Your Dietary Needs

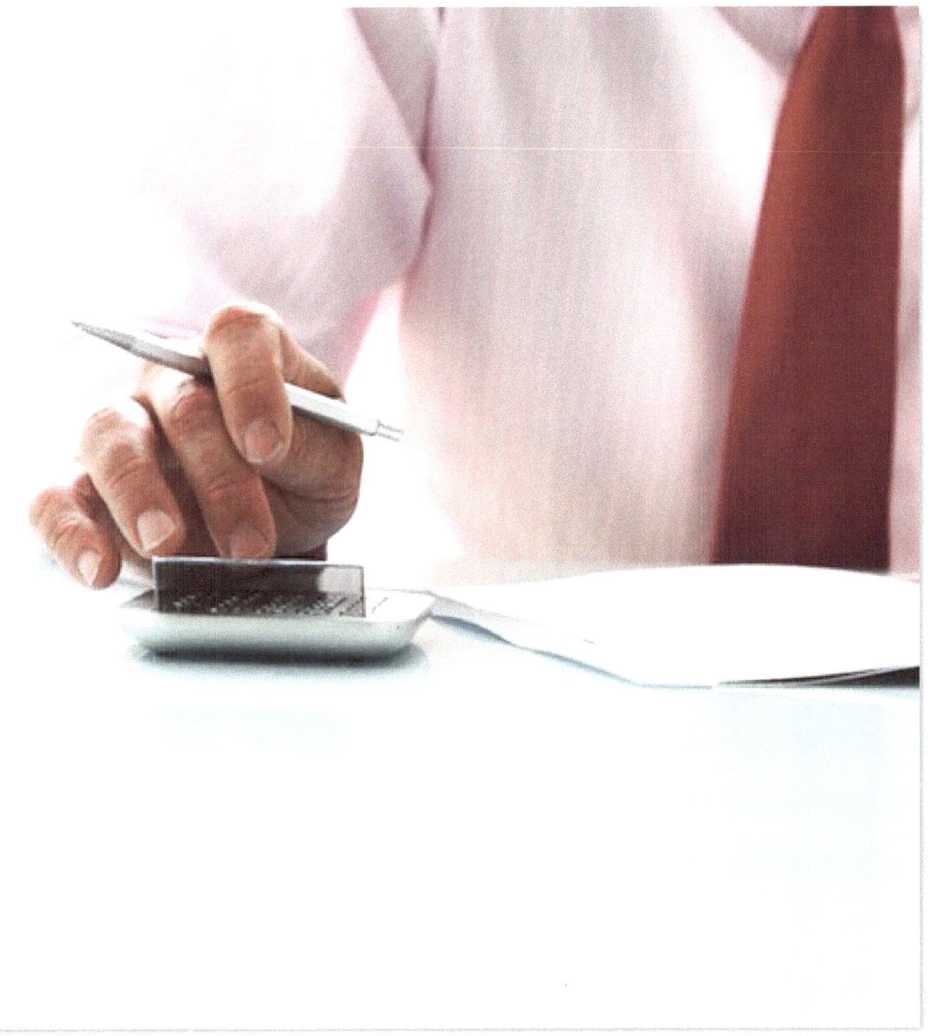

Many online tools offer a simple daily caloric needs calculator. Simply input your gender, age, height, weight, and activity level and the calculator produces a simple calorie estimate for the amount of nutrients you should aim to consume each day. Some calculators include BMI (body mass index) and BMR (basal metabolic rate) input sections as well, but not all.

A traditional calculation used by personal fitness trainers and dietitians suggests the following for calculating daily caloric needs:
Take your weight and multiply by 10 to get your RMR (resting metabolic rate). If you live a sedentary lifestyle, multiply this number by 10%; if moderately active then multiply by 20%; if active multiply by 30%. This second value is your DAB or Daily Activity Burn. Now add the RMR and DAB, and add the amount of calories you burn from exercise. If trying to lose weight, you would subtract the desired Calorie Deficit (usually about 500, but never more than 1000 unless under medical care) and the end-result is your daily target for calories consumed.

Weight x 10 = RMR

RMR x Lifestyle (10, 20 or 30%) = DAB

RMR + DAB + Calories Burned in Exercise = Daily Calorie Target

For weightloss:

RMR + DAB + Exercise - Deficit = Target

The United States Department of Agriculture offers a very nice Interactive DRI (Dietary Reference Intakes) calculator, pictured above, actually designed for healthcare professionals but fully accessible by all.

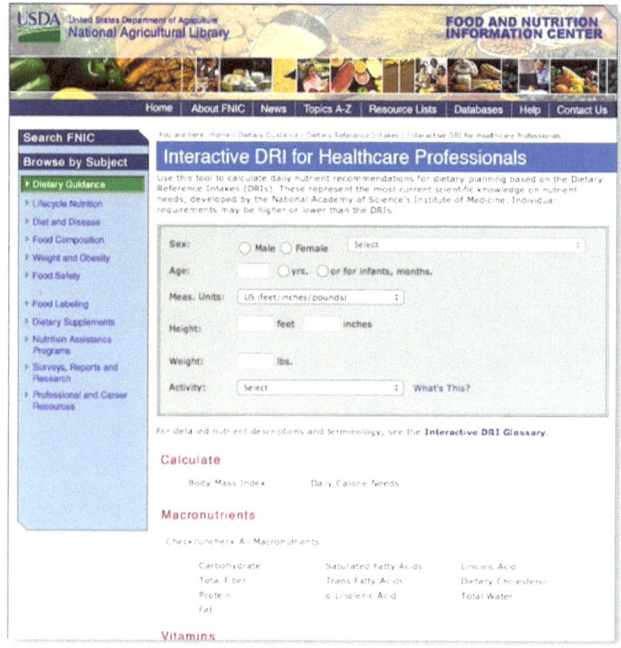

The calculator pictured here offers a simple approach to getting a healthy target for your daily caloric and nutritive needs.
http://fnic.nal.usda.gov/fnic/interactiveDRI/

Menu Planning

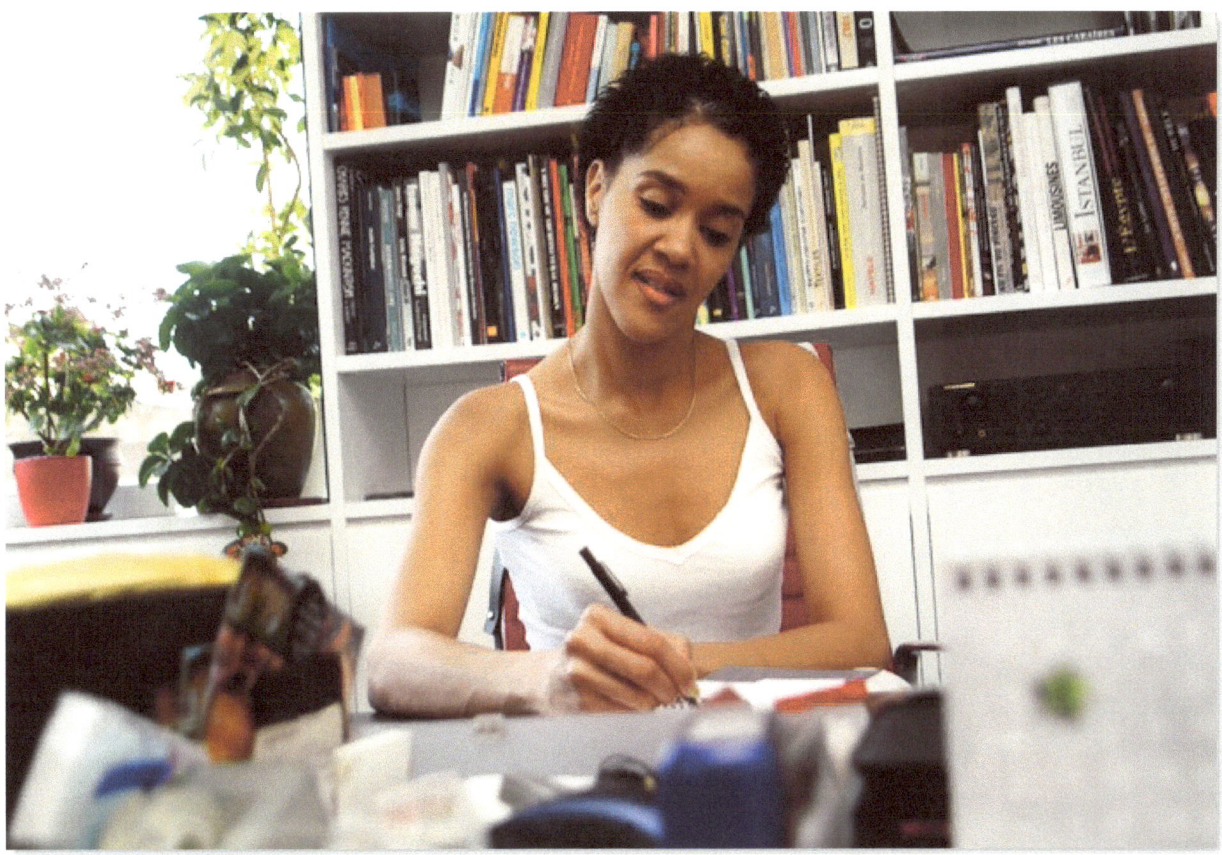

One of the smartest things I ever did was begin planning my menus in advance. By planning in advance, you do not need to calculate or track calories and nutrients every day. You also reduce the risk of grabbing less-than-healthy alternatives and straying from a health and fitness regimen because you don't have to think "what's for dinner?" you already have it written down.
In the previous section I offered several options for calculating a rough estimate of your daily caloric needs. That is a great place to begin your menu planning.

Let's say your caloric needs came out to 1600 calories per day, as an example. If you want to consume three full meals and two snacks, your menu may look like this:

Breakfast, Lunch, & Dinner 400 calories each

Two Snacks, 200 calories each

To keep my menus simple, I schedule two complete weeks of meals and snacks then repeat the two weeks 1-3 times to fill up a month or two. I do all the planning on paper with pens and pencils (and a calculator, if I don't have all the nutrition information for my recipes). Once I have two weeks scheduled, with three meals and two snacks for each day, I type up the menus in a template.

Microsoft Word and/or Excel have at least two free menu templates for this type of weekly meal plan:

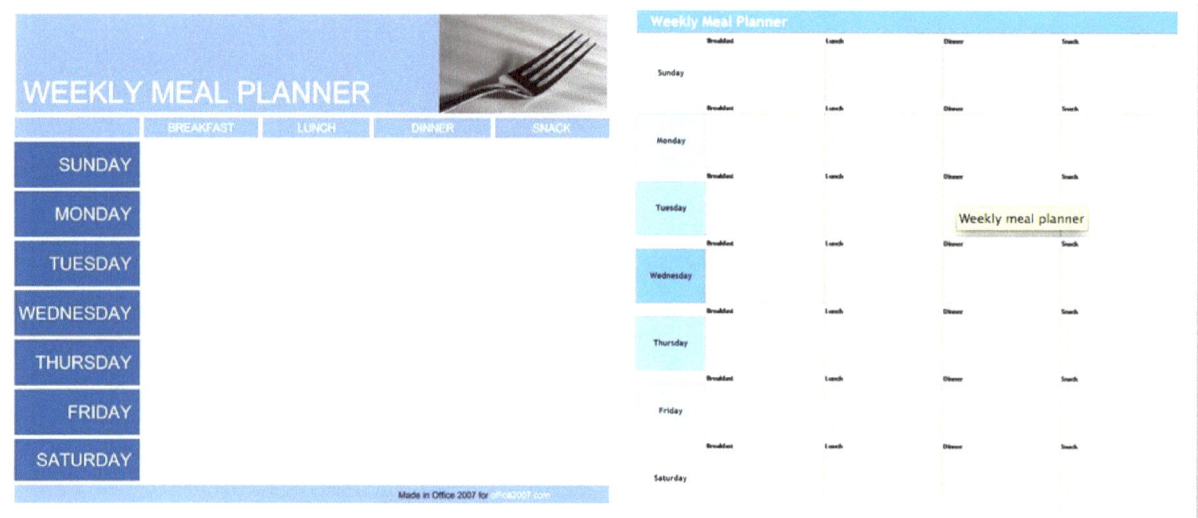

Screenshots from office.Microsoft.com

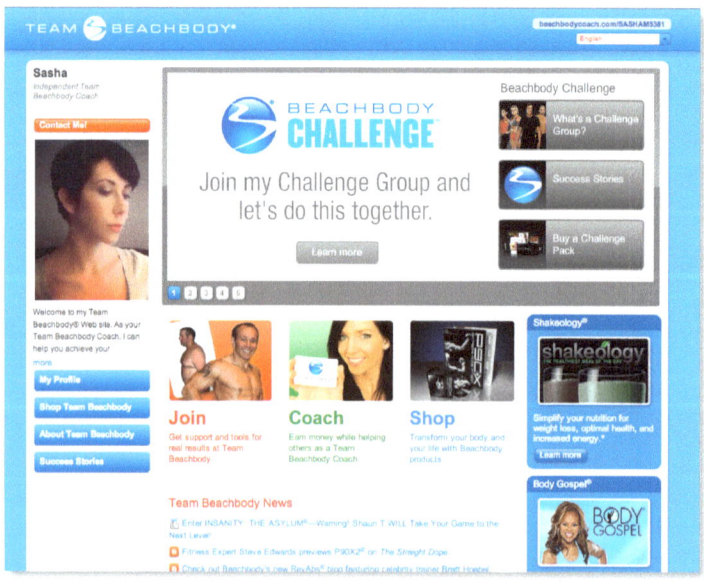

For personalized information and guidance on menu-planning and other health & fitness support, visit tinyurl.com/smaggio

Better Habits for Better Recovery

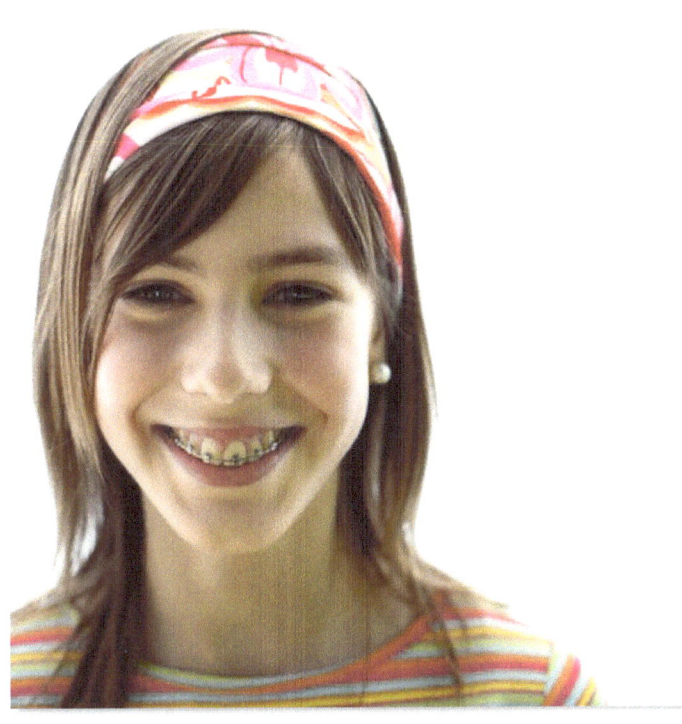

A commonly overlooked aspect of surgery preparation is pre-surgery nutrition and improving habitual behavior. As mentioned earlier, the longer you diligently care for your body before surgery, the greater the chances of a full recovery after surgery because you will bring your body closer to optimal health and throughout your recovery you will have an easier time ensuring proper nutrition, hydration, and rest.

Throughout this chapter I have presented very basic information on human nutrition and also provided tools and suggestions for improving your current pre-surgery nutrition and health efforts. There are a few things that do not fall into a simple category but I feel may help patients with their preparation efforts so I will present them here.

~ ~ ~ ~ ~ ~ ~ ~ ~ ~

Should I Gain Weight for Surgery?

Many patients facing jaw surgery worry about the liquid diet or no-chew diet they will need to consume during the initial 6 weeks, and possibly up to 12 weeks, following major jaw surgery. The thought of a liquid-only or no-chew diet is actually a deterrent for many patients - believe it or not, some people hear "liquid diet for 6 weeks" and they turn down the option for surgery. This should NOT deter you from having jaw surgery, especially if you have a malformation or other issue that can only be corrected with surgery, as in my case.

If the liquid-diet aspect doesn't get to the patient, the possible weightloss generally does. One of the most common questions I am asked is "How much weight did you lose after surgery?" The average patient loses about 10% of their starting bodyweight. If you currently weigh 160 lbs, then you can expect to drop up to 16 lbs during the first 6 weeks. Most of that weightloss occurs in the first 2 weeks because of the dramatic change in diet.

In my case, I lost about 8% of my starting bodyweight. I did not look sick or unhealthy, and I did not feel sick, unhealthy, weak, or nauseous. **The weightloss didn't concern me because I knew my body was getting enough nutrients to perform the tasks I needed, mainly recovering and maintaining health.**

As soon as possible, to improve your surgery and recovery process, I strongly urge you to assess your current health status and begin making small improvements. If you do not exercise at all, perhaps begin taking a 20-30 minute walk once a day or once every other day. If you have a dog, it's a safe bet the dog will appreciate the exercise too! If you don't have a dog, you could use the walk to listen to an audiobook or music, or you could offer to walk a neighbor's or friend's dog for company.

As far as gaining weight goes, it is more beneficial to improve your overall health before surgery by implementing some form of regular fitness or exercise, improving your nutrition and eating habits, drinking plenty of water, and improving your sleep.

Stop Skipping Meals

If you skip breakfast or skip lunch, now is the time to break this bad habit. People who tend to skip meals often begin feeling nauseous when they do eat them. If you have a tendency to skip breakfast or just have coffee, you may be familiar with that morning nausea that comes when you sometimes do eat breakfast. This WILL subside, and it will cease very quickly once you become consistent. The first few days of eating breakfast may leave you feeling a little sick throughout the morning, but before the end of the first week you will have countered this symptom of meal-skipping and actually begin enjoying breakfast.

Some people feel they just aren't hungry in the morning so they don't eat. This is another symptom of meal-skipping. Your body grows accustomed to the missed meals and releases dopamine, a neurotransmitter, to reduce hunger pangs and make you less hungry. There's a good chance you're slightly overweight if you do this, but there's an even better chance that you tend to choose less-healthy options at   lunchtime because of your sudden need to eat.

To help improve morning hunger, eat dinner before 7:30pm and refrain from eating after dinner. When you go to bed, you shouldn't be starving but you should feel like you're growing hungry. Drink a glass of water, at least 8-16oz, before bed to help nighttime hydration. This will also encourage easier waking the next morning because you will need to go to the bathroom!

Even if not hungry, try to consume breakfast within 60 minutes of getting up. If you're like me and prefer early morning workouts, then consume breakfast within an hour of completing your workout.

Visit Your General Doctor for a Checkup

Most people visit their general doctor or primary care physician (PCP) once a year for an annual physical exam. Schedule your next appointment with your doctor and make a list of questions or concerns you may have, including those regarding jaw surgery.

Any preexisting conditions or concerns regarding possible interference or complications with your surgery timeline MUST BE DISCUSSED AS SOON AS POSSIBLE. I stress this because during my research for my surgery I came across a video of a young lady prepared for surgery and the morning of her surgery she *only then* brought a possible concern to her surgeon regarding a family member that had an adverse reaction to general anesthesia. The result was her surgery getting canceled at the last minute and testing being scheduled. This is very expensive for hospitals and it's a selfish waste of time for you, your Team, and your surgical staff. **Don't be that patient that wastes people's time because you didn't ask questions when you had the opportunity to.**

During your physical exam, explain to your doctor that you are consulting with an OMF surgeon for corrective jaw surgery and you want to make sure that you are as healthy as you can be prior to that procedure. Ideally, your doctor will run a CBC (complete blood count) and check your red blood cells, particularly the hemoglobin and hematocrit (H&H), which will establish a current baseline for any possible current anemia. If your H&H are within normal range but on the lower end, adding a gentle iron supplement now can improve your recovery after surgery and reduce some of the difficult symptoms associated with anemia after surgery -- all those symptoms that I aggravated when I tried to push myself too soon.

I had my surgery on 13 December 2011 and I am completing this information playbook in January 2013, a little over a year later. Even now, I still take an iron supplement because after surgery I came to realize that my H&H were always low, but because they fell within the normal range it was never flagged by my lab work. After trying several varieties of iron supplements, I decided to stick with the **Ionic Iron liquid supplement by Trace Minerals.**

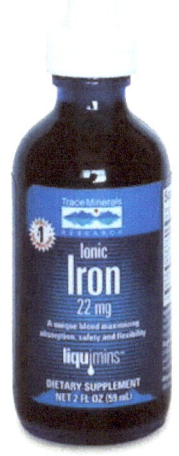

Photo from Trace Minerals

This iron comes with a dropper that has markings for the dose. I do not take the full recommended dose but instead only take about 0.5cc (1/2 milliliter). Even at this low dose, there are some digestive side-effects so to counter this I do occasionally add a Docusate gel capsule, especially if I have consumed foods that can produce constipation symptoms (e.g. cheese, too much fiber, etc.).

The CBC will also show your white blood cell count which will indicate general health or, if elevated, show signs of a possible infection or internal issue.

Journals

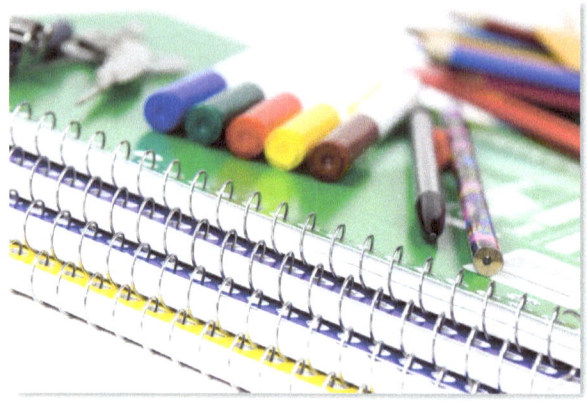

You can journal in a standard notebook or in a custom-designed food journal, available in most bookstores, health stores, online, and from tinyurl.com/smaggio

After surgery you will find it extremely helpful to keep a notebook or journal handy for writing down which medicine you take and when. It also helps to document your nutrition and water intake to make certain you're giving your body enough nutrients to work efficiently.

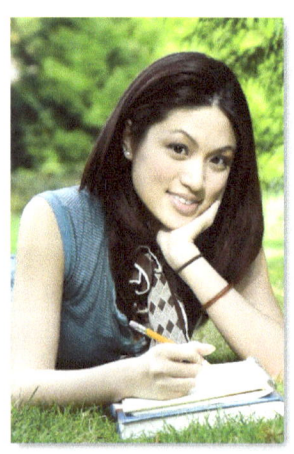

This seems like an easy "no-brainer" task but it's surprisingly difficult, especially if you're not accustomed to keeping track. As soon as possible, it is beneficial to get a notebook or food journal and begin tracking calories and specific nutrients, water, and exercise every day. Cholesterol is not an issue for me, personally, so I never track cholesterol, but I do track calories, protein, and fiber. I occasionally track sugar if I think I am consuming too much. I track my workouts and estimated calories burned (data gathered from a BodyMedia Armband) and I track water intake and sleep (from data also gathered from a BodyMedia Armband - www.bodymedia.com). During my recovery period, I tracked medicine by writing down what I took and when I took it so I could avoid taking too much or skipping doses.

I discuss this in greater detail in other Playbooks but I took a decongestant during the first week post-surgery, along with ibuprofen to prevent inflammation in the healing bones and tissue (different from swelling). I used saline and decongestant nose sprays, also for protecting my nose and sinuses from congestion, and I took antibiotics to prevent infection.

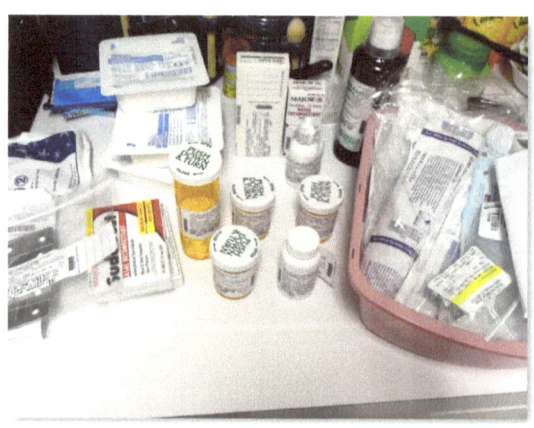

My bucket-o-medication that I was given when discharged from hospital after surgery

I was given more medicine than this but I didn't feel it was necessary. I was not in pain but took the ibuprofen as a precaution. If I didn't write the medicines and times down I would most certainly have forgotten because that first week, especially, was full of heightened anxiety. I wasn't very anxious after the surgery, I was actually more concerned with making sure I didn't forget anything important and that I consumed sufficient nutrients and water.

Don't Wait - Drink More Water Now

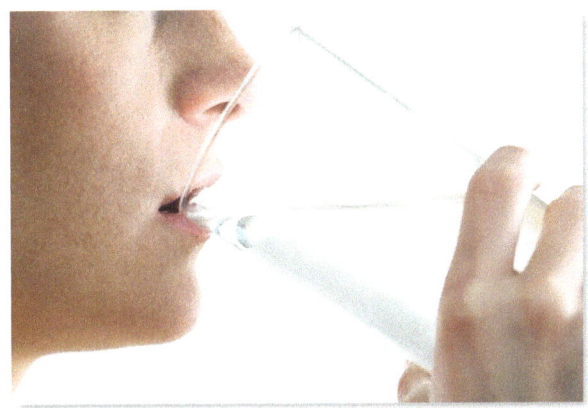

After surgery, one of the things they require before discharging you from the hospital is that you're demonstrating an ability and willingness to drink ample fluids on your own. In my case, my upper and lower jaws were bound shut with rubber bands so I was unable to open my teeth at all. This was uncomfortable but bearable. I had to use a syringe with a straw-like tube on the end and I had to slide the tube along my teeth and gums, positioning the end at the back of my teeth where my wisdom teeth had been. Then slowly depress the syringe to get the water behind my teeth and swallow.

I managed to do this without much trouble but I also had a strong determination to do more for myself. Some patients struggle with the syringe at first, so you must be patient.

Syringes aside, since they're irrelevant at this point, if you start consuming more and more water now you will have an easier time drinking plenty of water later. I have trouble drinking a lot of plain water. Many people do. It's plain. It's boring.

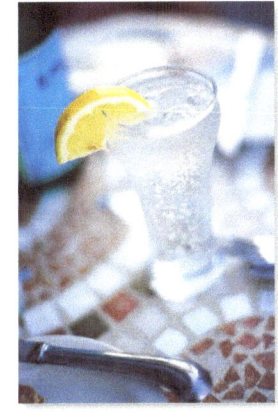

To make water more tolerable in large quantities I mix Truvia or other form of Stevia sweetener into my water along with either fresh lemon, fresh lime, or crystalized lemon or lime juice such as True Lemon and True Lime (www.truecitrus.com).

Improve Your Sleep

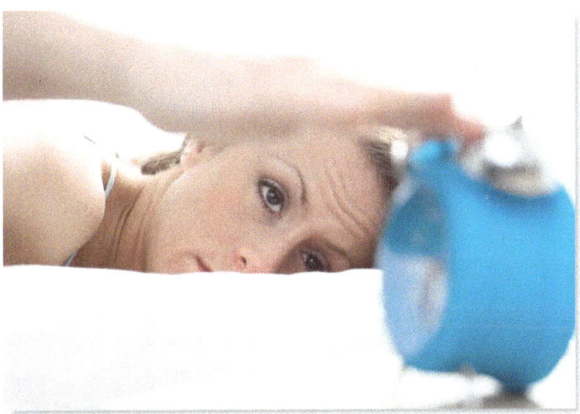

Improving your sleep before surgery will help with your body's ability to recover faster and more efficiently later. When we sleep, our brain has the ability to perform significantly more healing functions because we're not otherwise active. This is also the time when we're forming long-term memories which is a helpful tip for students - study then get a decent night's sleep!

It's difficult at first, but the best way I have found to improve sleep is to FORCE yourself up early. If you ever complained about having too few hours in a day, now is the time to make some more! Get up earlier than you normally have to. I prefer to wake up before the sun is up so I have the maximum amount of daylight hours each day for productivity. I also prefer to get my workout done during this time so it doesn't interfere with the rest of my day.

If you normally wake up at 7am, start waking up at 6:30am instead. Then after 1-2 weeks begin getting up at 6am. Drink a glass of cool water when you wake up to help refresh your body and rehydrate after sleep.

At the same time, each night begin going to bed about a half-hour before you normally would. If you normally go to bed between 11:30 and midnight, start getting ready at 10pm and lying down by 11pm. The goal is to arrange your sleep schedule for sufficient sleep while improving your ability to maximize each day.

You will find, over time, that a set amount of sleep is more comfortable for you. The recommended 8 hours each night is a bit much for me. I actually feel best when I sleep 5-7 hours and I maintained that 5-7 hours of sleep each night throughout my recovery after jaw surgery.

The forced sleep schedule will improve your body's functioning which will influence your healing rate. It will also affect your mood and energy levels in a positive way and improve your appetite.

Avoid napping. Napping interrupts your nighttime sleep so it's best to avoid them as much as you can. During your recovery, this will help reduce your swelling faster as well because the less time you spend lying down and asleep the more time you have for hydrating (drinking water) and consuming nutrients. Naps will actually make you feel more tired and more bored during recovery so the sooner you break this habit the better.

Improve Self-Care & Self-Sufficiency

You no doubt have tried internet searches for information and tips regarding jaw surgery and recovery, and in that search process you likely found many patients who complain about boredom during their recovery. Although I discuss the recovery process and experience in greater detail in other Playbooks, I will touch on the topic here since it's something you can work on improving and preventing now.

Boredom during recovery from jaw surgery generally stems from several factors. One major factor is a lack of self-care, which is more prominent in younger patients who live at home or are at home with parents and siblings during their recovery.

Self-care includes, but is not limited to, preparing your own meals, cleaning up when you're done preparing meals and eating, managing your own medicine, managing proper oral hygiene during recovery, and typical chores or tasks like laundry and light housework. **The more you do for yourself, the more you will feel in control of your situation and your recovery.**

Although you will feel tired during the first few days immediately after surgery, you should remember that there is nothing wrong with your arms and legs, or your brain, and you're fully capable of preparing food and serving yourself. The recipes in the Recipe Playbook will help serve as a guide for preparing your own recipes or you can simply use those. They include the exact same recipes I used for 6 weeks when I had major jaw surgery and they helped me prevent muscle loss (atrophy) and maintain health for better healing. I have since expanded the recipes to include many more, and divided them to suit liquid-only and soft-foods phases of recovery.

Begin preparing yourself mentally, even if your surgery is over a year away. You will want to get up and shower every morning during your recovery, if for no other reason than the steam helps with any nasal congestion and you will likely drool on yourself each night so showering refreshes you for a positive start to the day.

Even if you live at home with parents who want to do things for you, the sooner you work on doing more for yourself the easier your recovery will be. I don't live with my parents but my husband took the week off from work anticipating my need for assistance after surgery. The reality of the situation was that I really didn't need any help -- and this was a surprise for both of us.

Some things you can begin doing for yourself include laundry, especially if you don't do laundry now. This will give you something to occupy a little time during recovery and the light activity will make you feel productive, preventing boredom and mood swings. Helping with the dishes is also a great activity for jaw surgery recovery because it's simple and it doesn't require a lot of effort.

Not every home gets cluttered but mine does on occasion and **one thing I feel was a major benefit during my surgery preparation was cleaning and organizing my kitchen and bathroom.** I made sure the kitchen cupboards and pantry were organized so even if my face was very swollen I would be able to see, reach, and access everything I might need during cooking and food prep. I also cleaned and organized my bathroom.

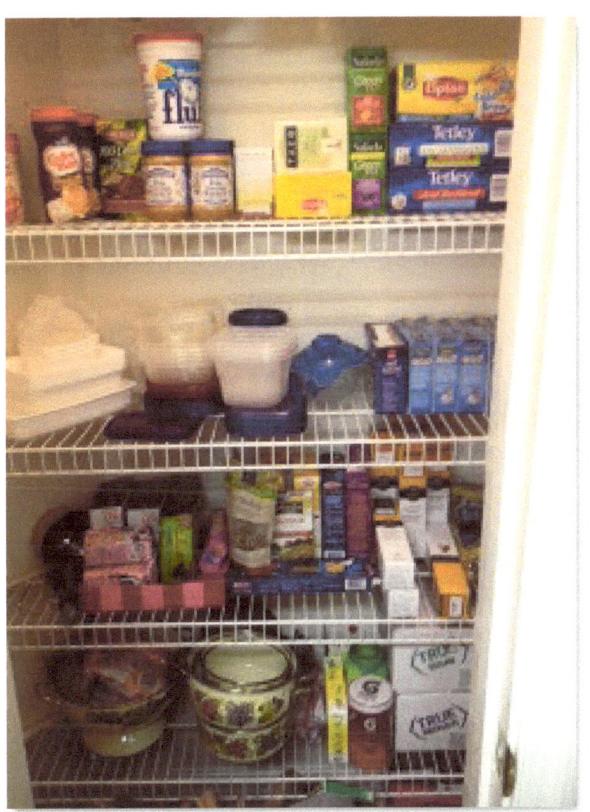

I organized my pantry closet, kitchen cabinets, spices, and storage containers before surgery so the stuff I knew I would want or need was easily accessible.

This made it much easier to put away my groceries when I had them delivered the day after I got home, and it made cooking and food prep much easier. Another helpful tip that would be a good habit to start now is rinsing dishes and cooking items as soon as you're done using them, and putting in the dishwasher. If you don't have a dishwasher, then wash them right away. **Nothing will be more frustrating than having to stand at the sink for 10-15 minutes washing dishes just to spend another 25-30 minutes preparing food that will take you a good 45-60 minutes to eat. Trust me!**

The first day home, I jumped in the shower, although I was bit drowsy from meds they gave me before discharging me at the hospital. It really helps to refresh your energy as soon as possible. I felt so much better once I could wash up and change, especially washing my hair because during the first week you have to wear a jaw bra (although this is mostly for lower-jaw surgery patients) and the jaw bra holds your hair really close to you scalp which makes it uncomfortable, but you get over it. The consequences of not wearing the jaw bra are deterrent enough to make you wear it (I discuss this in the Game Day and Recovery Playbook).

After I cleaned up and changed into clean clothes, I felt a lot better and more alert. I made a grocery list based on what I needed or wanted for the first week and I ordered the groceries using Peapod, a delivery service associated with Stop & Shop and Giant Supermarkets (www.peapod.com). If you have Peapod in your area, I highly recommend it for the convenience, especially right after surgery. If you don't have Peapod, you may have a local grocery delivery service available through your larger supermarkets.

I made two soups from recipes I had prepared in advance, but you'll learn from the other Playbooks that neither recipe worked with my syringes. That was disappointing and I was very frustrated because I hadn't eaten in almost two full days. I cleaned up though, after cooking, and made a calorie-rich hot cocoa with higher protein-content to tide me over [the recipe is in the Recipe Playbook] and I went to sleep by 10pm knowing my groceries would arrive around 6 o'clock the next morning and I'd be able to start fresh.

The point is, I was only one day post-surgery and even though I felt a little worn out and hungry (and ready to cry the moment I realized those soups were a waste of my time and energy), I did have sufficient energy to wash up and change, clean up the dishes my husband used the previous day while I was in the hospital (he would have cleaned them, but I didn't give him time). I made a grocery list, ordered groceries, cooked, cleaned up the dishes I'd used, and survived until a reasonable bedtime. I thought it best to avoid napping so my sleep would be better through that first night home.

Don't let the fact that it's MAJOR SURGERY influence your behavior.

You're still capable of doing PLENTY for yourself!

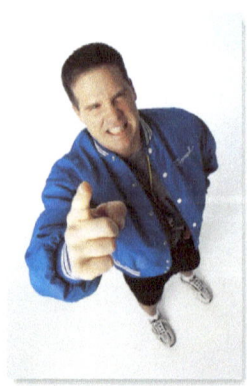

5
Patient Psychology

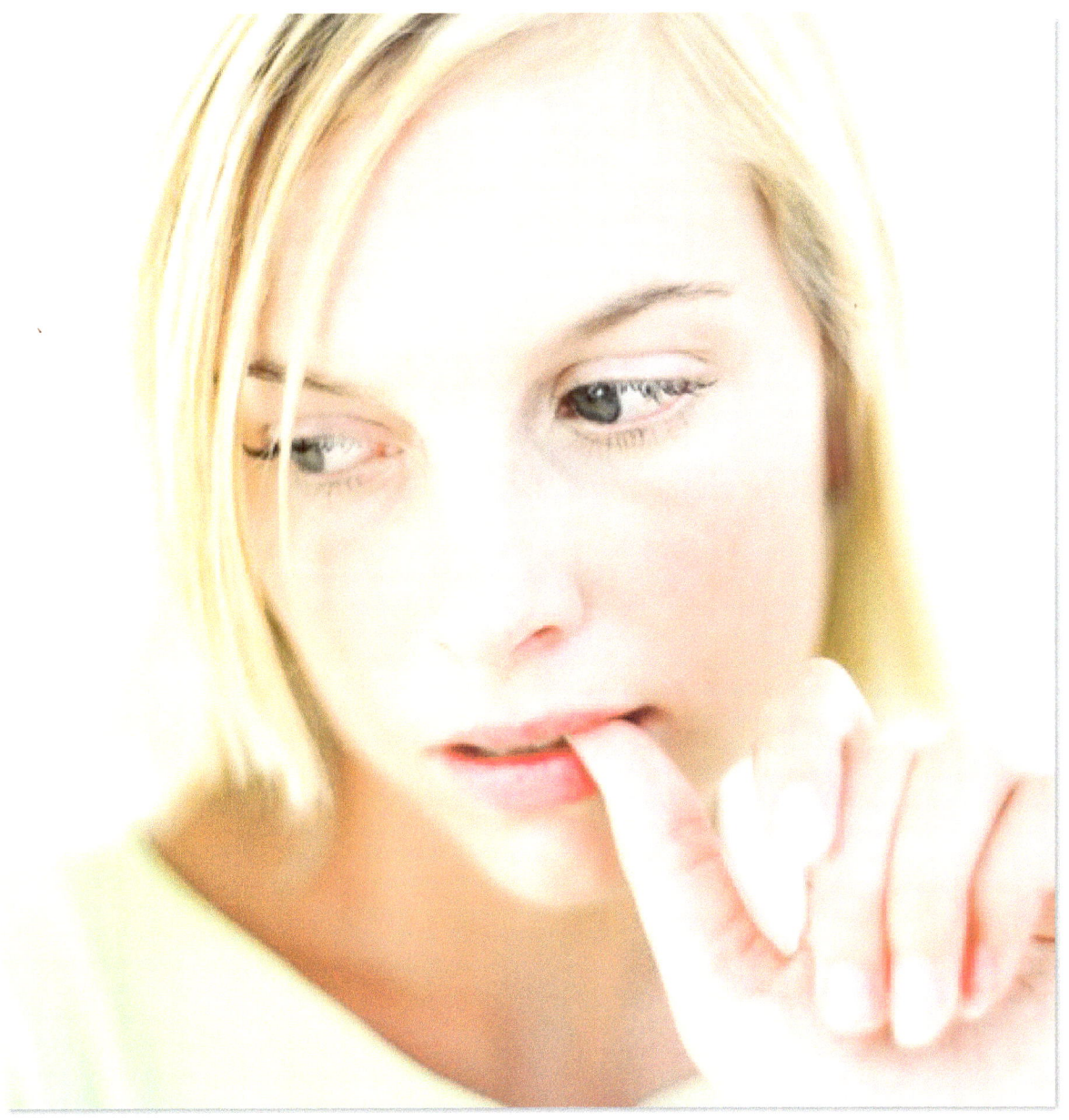

"Patient psychology is a major aspect of surgery and recovery, yet it's often overlooked by surgeons and patients." ~ Sasha

Mentally Preparing for Jaw Surgery

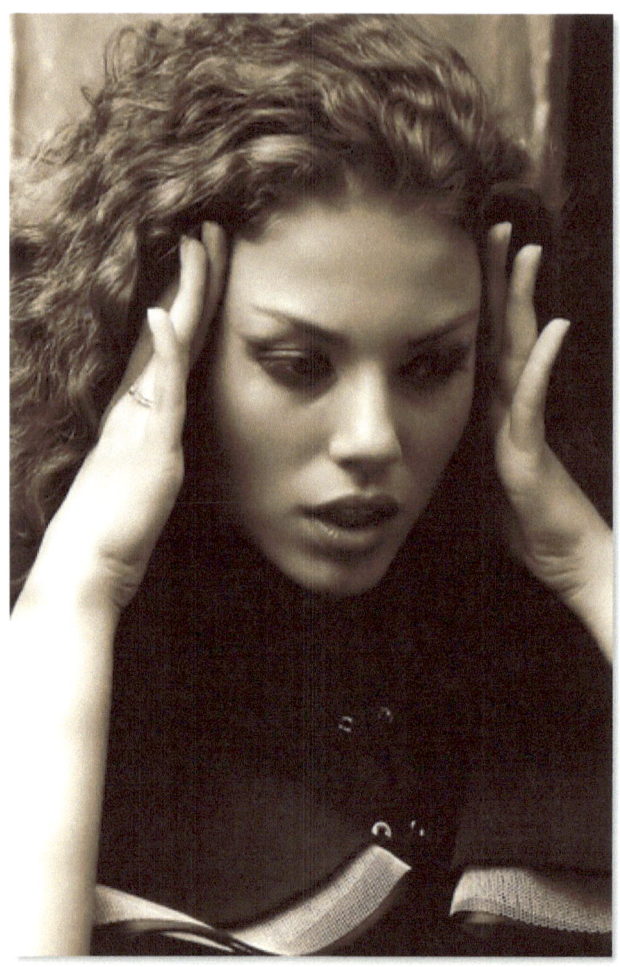

Preparing for corrective jaw surgery involves a great deal more than simply planning recipes for a liquid-only or no-chew diet. The psychological preparations for this type of surgery are just as important, if not more important, than the physical preparations.

You may have wondered if the jaw surgery will change the way you look, as many patients express concern regarding their appearance. Common questions presented to me by other patients include whether the surgery will change the way their nose looks; if surgery will make their face wider; if surgery will make their face look uneven or strange. These are only a few basic questions from a very long list, but these types of appearance or cosmetic questions are common from 99% of the jaw surgery patients that seek advice, tips, recipes, or support from me and the Jaw Recovery Playbook System.

~ ~ ~ ~ ~ ~ ~ ~ ~ ~

Organize Your Priorities

My best advice regarding the potential changes in physical appearance following corrective jaw surgery is: organize your priorities. There is always potential for changes to your appearance when the underlying bone structure is corrected, but don't lose sight of the fact that this is *corrective jaw surgery* which, in and of itself, implies that there is a problem with the current bone structure that requires some form of adjustment to function properly. This problem with the underlying bone structure, in many cases, has caused an asymmetrical appearance to the face which you, having grown accustomed to the asymmetry, may feel is a "normal" appearance for you. The surgery will improve symmetry for a better physical appearance as a minor goal behind the primary goal of improving overall functionality.

Consider it this way: if your bones had grown (or stopped growing) at the ideal moments throughout your life, your facial

features would have adjusted to the natural symmetry formed. **The jaw surgery is, ideally, restoring symmetry that should have been present had your bones grown the way they are naturally expected to. If your bones had grown as expected, there would be no need for surgery.**

Your surgeon will work to improve your appearance - not to make it worse. Everything the surgeon does is working toward an end-result in which you are happy with not only the improved functioning of the upper and lower jaws, but also happy with improved quality of life and improved physical appearance, ensuring your overall happiness with the experience.

Although I discuss this in greater detail in the Game Day and Recovery Playbook, even a year after my jaw surgery I still look at myself in pictures or in the mirror and have to adjust the way I hold or angle my head and face before I'm comfortable with what I see. It's not 'bad' but it's an adjustment that takes time. **Try not to confuse your 'adjustment period' with dissatisfaction or unhappiness; they are not the same thing.** Some patients finally feel 100% comfortable around the 2-year mark, so give it time and expect to give it time.

No One is to Blame for This

Especially with younger patients, blaming is sometimes common. "If my parents did [this], I wouldn't have needed surgery." Even in my case, I wore braces for two years as a teenager and I still required braces a second time and major surgery to correct my occlusion. I asked my surgeon, "If the braces had been done properly when I was kid, would the need for surgery have been prevented?"

He assured me that would never be the case. In my case with apertognathia, I had an open-bite but overall my genes just didn't trigger the appropriate amount of growth at the right times to ensure my upper and lower jaws fit nicely as needed for facial symmetry and functionality. This caused problems with the way my upper and lower jaws came together (the occlusion) and was further exacerbated with a tongue-thrust issue that likely would not have developed had my teeth met in the right spots to begin with. There was no "one thing" that caused the problems for my jaws, it was a number of things that worked together to undermine my overall functioning.

It's important, however, to remember this is no one's fault. **The fact that jaw surgery is an option should be welcomed and appreciated; not an opportunity to place arbitrary blame.** Patients whose parents express concern that they may be at fault should be reassured that the problems were created and controlled at a genetic level and nothing they could have done as parents would have prevented the need for surgery.

There are, of course, a few exceptions such as cases where the problem stems from injury but generally - **when I refer to corrective surgery here, and throughout the Jaw Recovery Playbook System, I am referring to cases of natural malformations resulting in an uncontrollable situation that requires surgery to fix.**

Managing Stress

We all get stressed. Jaw surgery patients are no different from the everyday person going through a stressful time. How we manage our stress will ultimately define how we feel throughout and about the experience, but it will also influence the way those around us respond to our behavior, emotions, and needs.

How willing to help someone else would you be if they did nothing but complain, whine, and act in a negative manner? It's really difficult to want to help that type of person, but it's even more difficult for many of us to see ourselves objectively and catch that type of mindset and behavior in advance.

The same goes for working with your orthodontist and surgeon. They may be paid to perform services for you, but you will have far more pleasant an experience working with them if you treat them with respect and appreciation. If your surgeon is a Resident at a teaching hospital, like mine was, then your initial encounters may seem chaotic and confusing which make the scary jaw surgery experience even more difficult to manage. If I had known from the beginning that the hospital I was going to is a teaching hospital, I could have adjusted my attitude from Day One which would have reduced my frustration with my surgeons after being turned away three times and told I wasn't quite ready yet.

Some patients have expressed concern to me about having a Resident perform their surgery, when I recommend they check out nearby teaching hospitals. To clear up the misunderstanding, **Residents are not pulled out of class, stuck in the operating room with a jaw surgery patient, and given free reign of the procedures.** I tell everyone that asks me how to find a good surgeon for jaw surgery, *"Find your nearest teaching hospital with a good reputation and see if they will perform your surgery there."* This is because you will have not one surgeon but a TEAM of OMFS Residents working together to improve your surgery experience with plenty of oversight from experienced surgeons. This also reduces frustration some patients have reported to me from working with a stubborn older surgeon who might be set in his or her ways following out-dated or less-efficient methods.

Moreover, teaching hospitals are sometimes significantly easier to get coverage at for expensive procedures because you're essentially serving in a "practice" role for the Residents, even though the entire experience is well-organized and guided by experienced surgeons. You're doing a little bit of good for OMFS Residents while getting quality care in return.

Food for thought: I think that it's easier to be patient with Residents than surgeons with years of experience because you see the Residents as surgeons-in-training and you want to shape their experience to help them become excellent providers for their future jaw surgery patients. On the other hand, I'm also the type of person to head straight to the "Cashier-in-Training" register at the grocery store because I know I can be patient with the new cashier and my patience will help shape the cashier's experience while in training.

Improving your understanding of the surgeon's side of things can help influence the way you approach these visits with your surgeon and surgical team. You have a lot of control in this situation, which I will discuss next, you simply have to take responsibility for yourself and your treatment. This will greatly reduce the negative aspect of stress throughout your surgery process and the better you manage your stress, the better your Team will be able to assist in your recovery and the better your Offensive Coordinators will be able to guide your treatment.

How to Deal with Stress

You will have trouble accepting this, but the best way to manage stress of ANY KIND is to exercise regularly, eat right, drink plenty of water, and sleep on schedule. Life is full of stress and stressors - that's a fact and no one will ever deny it. Stress affects the body in a number of physiological ways which can lead to headaches or migraines, poor sleep, chronic aches and pains, poor appetite, and frequent illness. Stress weakens our immune systems making it easier for us to get sick and making it more difficult to get rid of common colds. But you can control this and improve the way your body handles stress by giving it the right tools to work with.

Let's say you're tasked with building a table, but you're only given wood and nails. You have no hammer, no measuring devices, no saw or cutting tools, and no instructions. How well do you think that table will turn out? Your body is the same with the tasks you give it.

You want to avoid getting sick, but you don't give your body any tools to work with. You want to lose weight or look more toned and defined, but you don't give your body the tools to get those results. You want to be at your absolute healthiest by the time you reach your jaw surgery date, but you're not giving your body any help.

Bodies are extremely smart and very resilient. If you give your body the tools it needs, it can do almost anything. Your body will do the things you ask of it as long as you give it what it needs to function at its best.

These tools are:

- **WATER** - essential for all internal functions but sufficient hydration will also reduce dry skin and dry lips, dry eyes, frequent headaches, and a variety of other common issues.

- **NUTRITION** - not just food and calories, but quality ingredients for balanced nutrient intake. Sufficient protein, fiber, and vitamins while reducing sugar and sodium intake.

- **EXERCISE** - improved digestion, metabolism, physical appearance, posture, reduces aches and pains, and improves sleep.

If fitness and nutrition have not been a major part of your life before now, there is no time like the present to begin improving your health.

There are a number of free online resources for fitness and nutrition support.

Bodybuilding.com offers complete workout regimens for free. Most of the workout plans include some general nutrition guidelines to help maximize results and most workout programs through Bodybuilding.com include daily worksheets to track the amount of weight used and the number of repetitions.

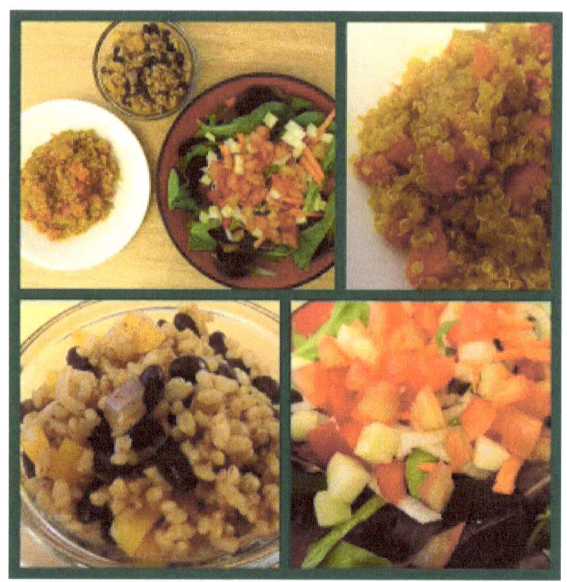

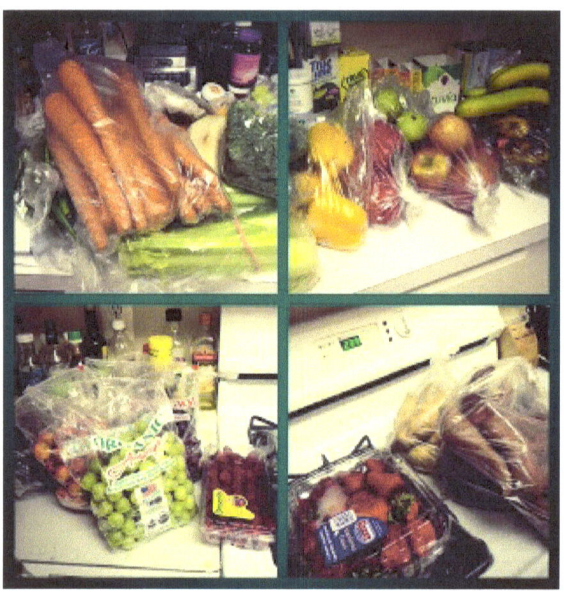

© Photos by Sasha Maggio

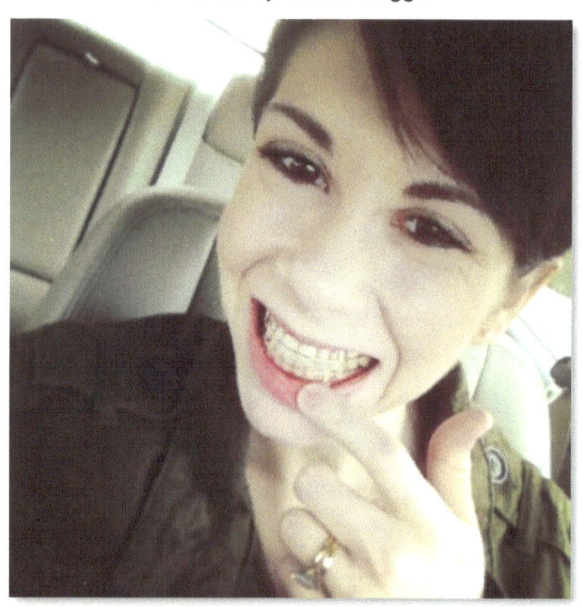

I offer personalized nutrition and fitness coaching through Beachbody, a major manufacturer of top-selling home fitness programs. It's not a full-time position but I help any who wish to improve their health and fitness through consistent, manageable effort. The Beachbody resources are available for residents of the U.S. and Canada, including U.S. territories, but access may be limited for international clients. Check out tinyurl.com/smaggio for more information.

As a health and fitness coach, I provide helpful tips, tools, and support for menu planning, shopping, food prep, recipes, and exercise.

Food Journal from
tinyurl.com/smaggio

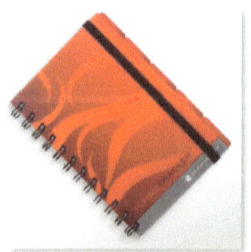

Finding Control

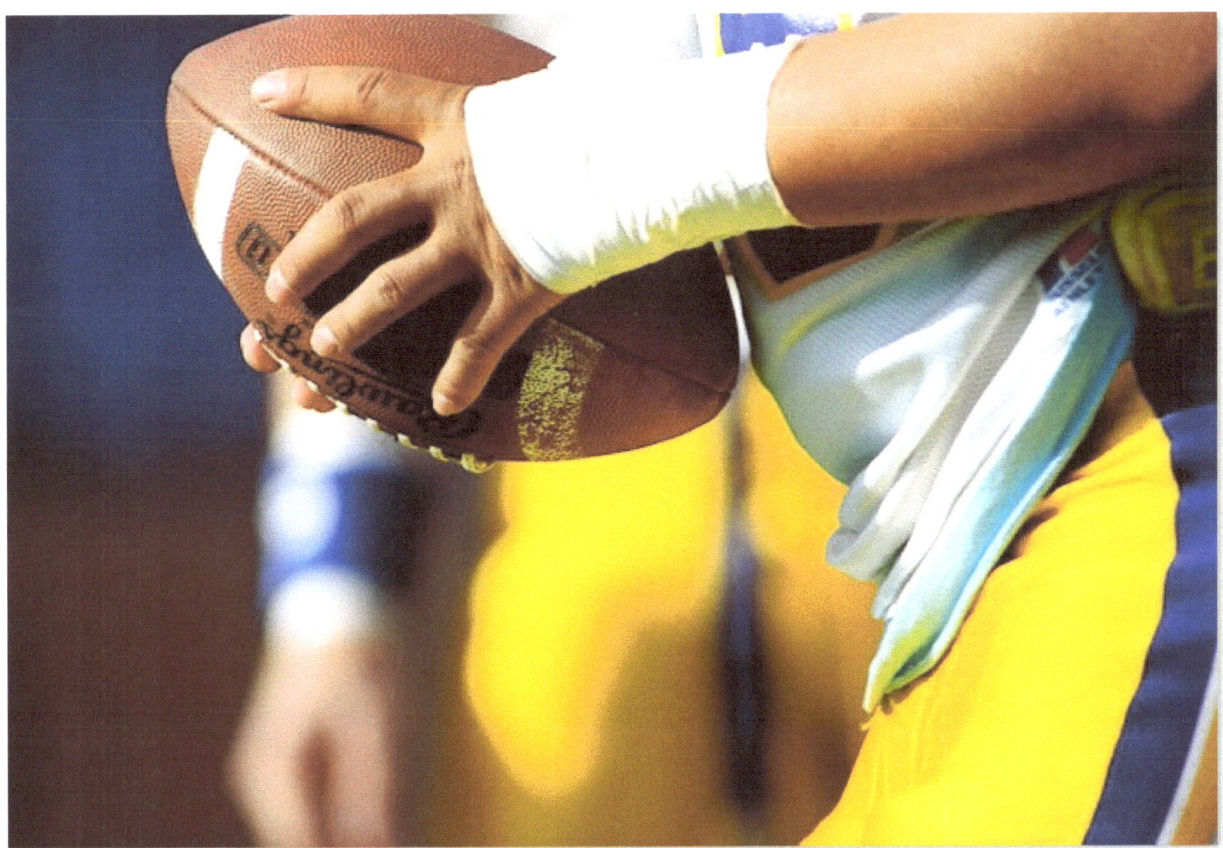

As mentioned many times throughout this Playbook, **you actually have all the control in your surgery experience, you simply have to accept responsibility for it.** Younger patients living at home with parents often fall into the habit of leaving their treatment, appointments, and surgery plans up to their parents. This creates frustration and both the patient and the parents are usually quite agitated by the time they come to the Jaw Recovery Playbook for support.

The **Defense Playbook** offers helpful resources, tips, advice, and support for parents, and other caregivers involved in the patient's surgery and recovery processes.

This, however, is the **Offense Playbook** in which the advice and guidance is generally meant for the patient.

As the patient, **YOU** are your **OWN** Quarterback. **YOU** control the situation. **YOU** guide **YOUR** Team to best suit **YOUR** needs. No one else can do this for you.

If you attempt to leave the control in the hands of others, you will almost certainly feel stressed out, frustrated, misunderstood, and out of control <u>throughout the entire</u> process.

Regardless of age, you (the patient and Quarterback) can take control by taking responsibility for yourself and your treatment. This is NOT your mother's surgery, or your father's surgery. This is not your husband's surgery or your wife's surgery. This is **YOUR** surgery - **OWN IT!**

Taking Control of Your Treatment

The best way to take control of your jaw surgery treatment is to follow the guidance listed throughout this book. Make your own appointments with your orthodontist and your surgeon or surgical team. Attend the appointments with a notebook so you can write down the information as it is said to you. This way you won't forget, because you don't have to remember; it's written down. This will simplify the explanation process as you relay information from your surgeon and orthodontist to the other members of your Team.

Use the notebook to write down your questions as you think of them. Also write down concerns you may have, even if not in the form of questions, so you have a list to improve communication with your surgeon at your appointments.

Consider how often you stress out. If you're a student or work full-time, this might be more often than not. You will want to control your appointment scheduling so you are not also being stressed from exams, mid-terms, projects due, or temporary business/work tasks. The stress from these everyday-life situations will affect your ability to focus at your appointments and the stress will make you feel rushed or in a hurry, so long appointments with your surgeon will likely result in a lot of frustration and possibly emotional outbursts. This is true for patients of all ages and genders, so don't feel like there's any restriction on your feelings.

Take Control of Your Attitude

By managing your own treatment and improving your health and fitness with regular exercise and a proper diet, you will have an easier time controlling your attitude. Don't misunderstand, however, because by controlling your attitude I am **not** implying that any frustration or emotions you feel you must hide.

You are entitled to feel frustrated when things keep changing and you're unsure of what's going on. But you can control this and actually reduce frustration by improving communication between yourself and your surgeon, and also improving communication between your surgeon and orthodontist.

By writing down notes at your surgical appointments, you will have better information to share with your orthodontist. It's not entirely up to you, though. **Do not hesitate to pressure your surgeon to communicate clearly and effectively with your orthodontist if you feel that they are not working on the same page.** Likewise, do not fail to trust your surgeon is doing everything possible even if it seems that you're standing still rather than progressing. Sometimes, you just have to be a little more patient.

In my situation, my surgical team was at a military hospital and my orthodontist was a civilian. The surgeons in the military operate in a slightly different manner from civilian surgeons so the communication lines between my orthodontist and surgeons were not clear throughout the first 8-12 months of my orthodontic treatment. This, combined with the fact that I was not entirely aware that the hospital is a teaching hospital, set me up for a significant amount of frustration which led to some emotional outbursts, tears, irritability, and negativity after nearly every appointment in the beginning. **None of this was productive at all!**

Once I realized where the problem was, I pressured my surgeon to make time to contact my orthodontist and actually TALK so they were clear on what needed to be done in order to get me ready for surgery. I also adjusted my attitude toward my surgeon and his team because I was then aware that it is a teaching hospital and their experience with me could affect the way they work with other patients. I wanted to improve their experience just as much as I wanted to improve my own.

If something is unclear - <u>ASK</u>

If something is bothering you - <u>ASK</u>

If you think there's a miscommunication somewhere between your surgeon and your orthodontist - <u>ASK</u>

If you don't speak up, you have no right to feel frustrated or irritated by the outcome and you certainly cannot complain about the way the surgeon and orthodontist operate if you don't care enough about your own treatment to step up and take control.

Dealing with Others

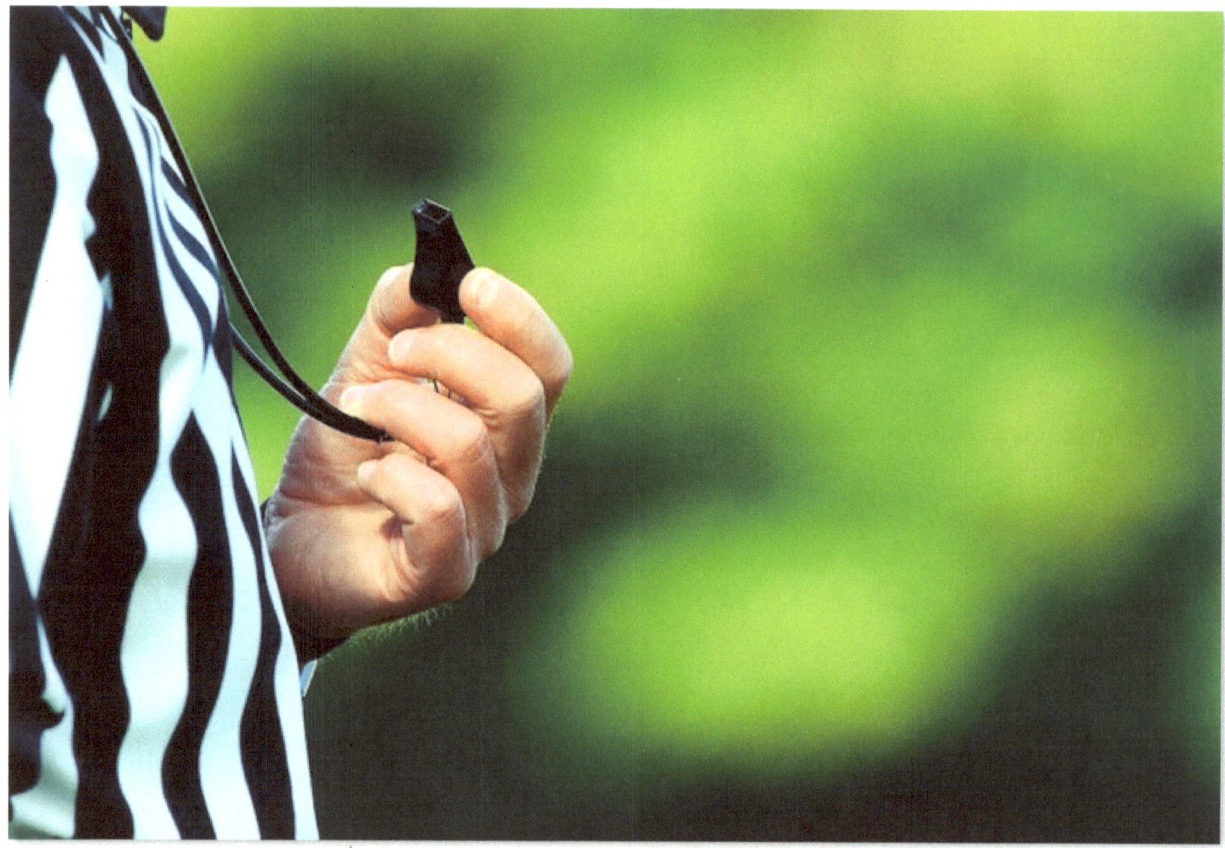

Apart from the fact that orthognathic surgery is a major surgery to deal with, and the treatment process is longer than many patients expect due to the unpredictable pace of orthodontic treatment, a major obstacle many jaw surgery patients face is unexpected opposition.

When we tell others that we are going to have jaw surgery, one of the most common reactions is, "You look fine to me, I don't think you need surgery." It doesn't help, does it? It certainly didn't help me when I was dealing with anxiety over my upcoming surgery.

People who do not have jaw or occlusion issues have a difficult time understanding why something that seems so extreme is so necessary. No matter how you try to explain it, they just cannot grasp what it's like to have trouble speaking simply because your lower jaw never lines up the same way twice as you open and close your mouth, or trouble with a lisp or speech impediment from an open-bite or other malocclusion.

They have trouble understanding what it's like to bite into food and only be able to chew with the teeth in the back of your mouth. Open-bite patients like me often have trouble with even soft foods because we can't bite with the front teeth. I can't count the times I had to bring a napkin to my face to hide my mouth as I attempted to adjust food after trying to bite into a sandwich or burger only to pull back and leave all the toppings hanging from the bread, or worse, hanging from my mouth. It was so embarrassing!

It was embarrassing to the point where I didn't feel comfortable dining at a restaurant and if I did go out to eat I would have to avoid all the food items I wanted and order something I knew I could cut up and eat with a fork. Eating pizza with a knife and fork is just not the same…

Some patients have trouble with sleep apnea or breathing, chronic congestion, and a host of other troubles all stemming from the jaw alignment issues. Non-patients have a hard time understanding all of this.

When we say, "jaw surgery" non-patients hear "cosmetic surgery" and instantly think we are doing this for appearance reasons. While some patients benefit from the aesthetic aspects of corrective jaw surgery, many do not have any physical appearance changes at all.

For my surgery, I was originally scheduled for a 3-piece Le Fort I and a Bilateral Sagittal Split-Osteotomy (BSSO). A Le Fort I refers to the cut along the upper jaw that runs behind the nose and above the roots of the top teeth. The "3-piece" part refers to the dividing of the upper jaw (along the palate) into three sections in order to reshape the upper jaw for a better fit. The BSSO is a sort of angled cut at the sides (bilateral) of the lower jaw and then the front portion of the lower jaw is slid forward to improve alignment, and often profile as well.

At the last minute, my surgery was changed to a 3-piece Le Fort I (same as planned) and genioplasty (instead of the BSSO). Genioplasty is a very common cosmetic procedure, though, so I sometimes get more comments about that as if the procedures were entirely elective. While they were elective - no one forced me to have surgery - the basic truth is that if I didn't have surgery I would never have a proper bite/alignment. Braces alone could never fix my problem. While the genioplasty helped balance my profile, it was not actually "necessary" in the functional sense. It was, however, necessary to improve the symmetry after adjusting the upper jaw so dramatically.

If the original BSSO procedure had been performed, it would have been wasted effort because the changes to the positioning and angle of my upper jaw allowed the two jaws to meet properly without moving the full lower jaw. Instead of moving the full lower jaw, which would have moved my teeth too, the surgeon simply moved my chin to adjust my profile.

Honestly, it could have been more dramatic, but I'm satisfied with the results I received.

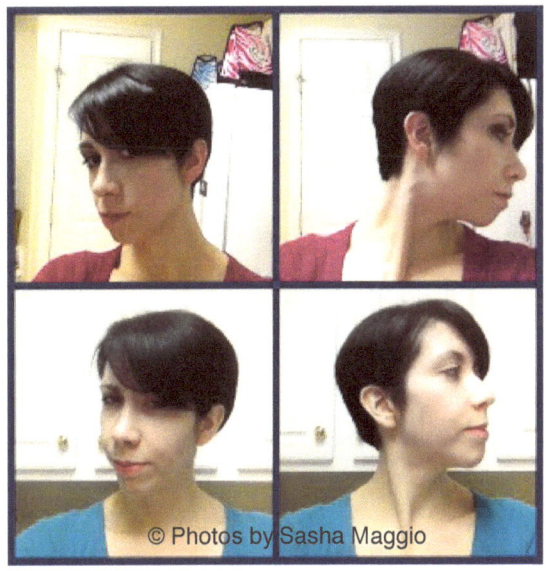
© Photos by Sasha Maggio

Expectation Management

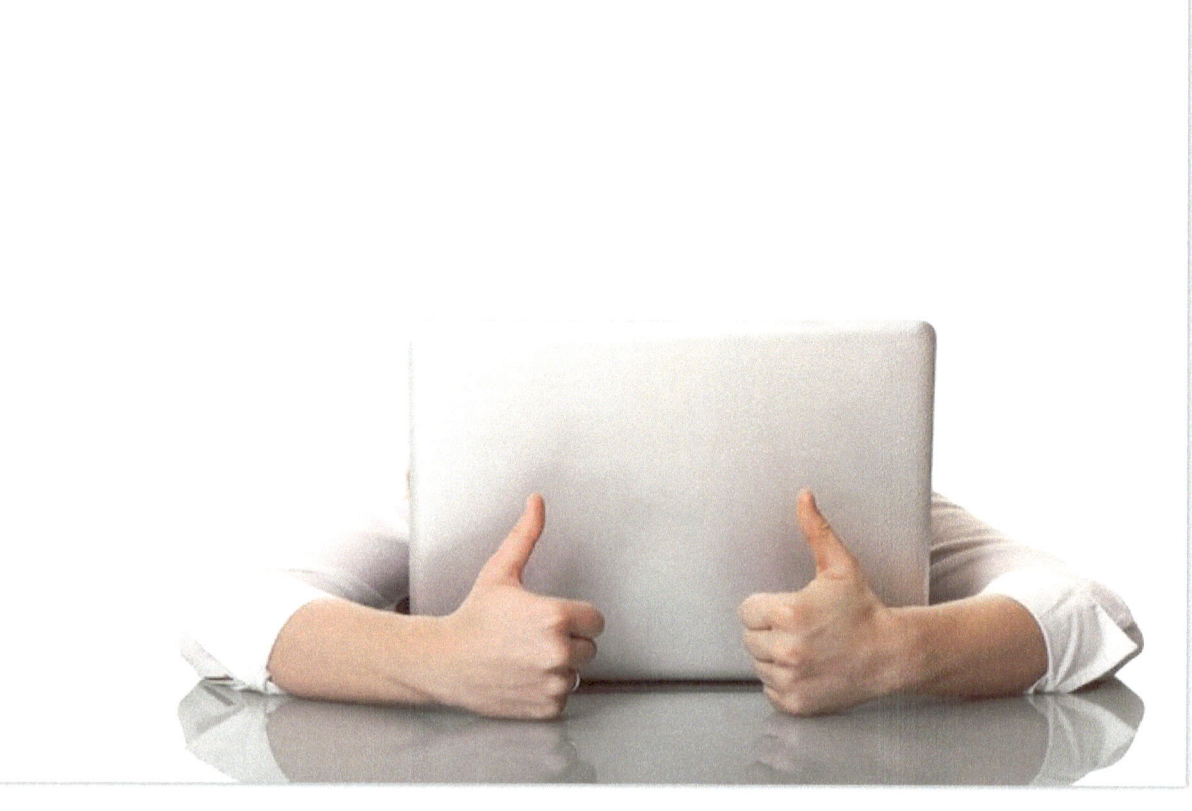

As mentioned, **one of the most frustrating aspects of the entire orthodontic and jaw surgery process is waiting.** Much of the timeline consists of waiting. Waiting for your next orthodontist appointment. Waiting for the braces to move your teeth into position for surgery. Waiting for the surgeon to say you're ready. Eventually waiting for surgery and then waiting some more for your recovery to be complete (or complete "enough") for your orthodontist to complete your braces. Then you have to wait until your teeth are properly situated and the braces can come off but you learn it's not over because now you've got years of retainers ahead of you.

It really seems like a never-ending process and **at the beginning it can seem like you will never be surgery-ready.**

I know -- I was in that boat too.

Other frustrations arise when the patient doesn't understand something about their treatment or the treatment process. I experienced this also; for example, three times my orthodontist sent me to the surgeons believing I was ready for surgery and each time I spent well over an hour (sometimes several hours) in the OMFS department while the surgeons and Residents took x-rays, impressions, pictures, and measurements only to tell me I wasn't quite ready yet. Each time it seemed as if something new was popping up that the surgeons hadn't mentioned before, to the orthodontist or to me, which demonstrated an issue in their communication lines and also an issue in my management of my own treatment.

Expectation Management

Expectation management is a logical approach to situations in which we do not have all the control so we cannot clearly predict the outcome or timeline. For example, at my initial consult for surgery before my braces were applied, the surgeon said I should be ready for surgery in about 6-8 months once the braces are put on. If I had assumed this was an accurate timeline prediction, I would have been extremely disappointed when 6-8 months rolled around and I was still not ready. I wasn't ready at 12 months or 14 months either. To prevent disappointment, at least to some degree, I actively tried to refrain from expecting surgery any time before 12 months. This active thought process is a type of "expectation management" to help reduce the negative effect of unmet expectations.

When my surgery was complete, I was told I had to wait at least 6 weeks before the archwires could be replaced and my orthodontics treatment could continue to completion. In reality, I went to see the orthodontist early because a bracket had come loose and I wanted him to check my progress. Then at 6 weeks I went to see him again to have my archwires replaced after my bite-splint was removed. The bite-splint held my teeth in place despite the cut archwires from my 3-piece procedure, but this is discussed in greater detail in the Game Day and Recovery Playbook. At that time, my orthodontist explained that it should be 3 months or so before the braces would be ready to come off. Not much work had to be done, there were just a few minor adjustments still needed. **A year after surgery, my braces were still on.** Thirteen months after surgery, my braces were still on. By that point, my ability to maintain my expectation management was waning, but knowing they would be finished soon, I worked hard to continue my treatment with a positive attitude. They were finally removed at a little over 13 months post-surgery.

It seems so simple, but keep in mind that it requires practice and continued effort.

Tips for Expectation Management

- **The type of braces will affect your treatment timeline.** Traditional braces are the slowest option. For most jaw surgery patients, Invisalign and Lingual Braces are not options because the brackets and wires must be on the front surfaces of the teeth for surgery. **Self-ligating braces** tend to reduce treatment time. Consider all options before making your decision.

- **If your orthodontist suspects you need corrective surgery to complete your treatment, it is usually best to consult with a surgeon before having your braces put on (if possible).** Some insurance companies are particular about the way orthodontics treatment and corrective jaw surgery are billed and you may need to go back and forth with your health insurance (NOT dental insurance) to ensure coverage of your surgery. If your braces are put on first, and the insurance process takes 18 months before you have full approval, you may be left with braces for well over 2 years before you're ready for surgery.

- **In many cases, for upper-jaw surgery, the teeth are moved into an awkward position before surgery so they line up properly afterward** and this is another reason to hold off on braces until you are sure of the insurance situation for surgery. In my case, my open-bite was made significantly worse to the point where I had to strain in order to close my lips over my teeth and I could only effectively chew with about 4 teeth in the back of each side of my mouth. I would not have wanted to prolong that while waiting for insurance paperwork.

- **Your orthodontist can only move your teeth as quickly as the teeth are willing to be moved in a safe manner.** Pressuring the orthodontist to move your teeth faster may be asking the impossible, depending on the type of braces you have.

- **Your surgeon cannot approve you for surgery until your mock-surgery demonstrates a positive result.** The mock-surgery is very simple to understand - the surgeon has impressions made of your upper and lower teeth then creates a model of the two sets of teeth to demonstrate your current bite or alignment. The surgeon will then perform a mock-surgery in which he cuts or repositions the upper and lower teeth in the way he will during your surgery to see how they line up when finished. If the result can be improved, you will have to wait a bit longer. I did this three times!

- **The hardest part of surgery for most patients is the time leading up to the surgery itself.** The recovery period is often a lot easier than people realize or expect, but expecting a difficult recovery can help improve your recovery experience. A friend of mine underwent similar double-jaw surgery a year before I did and her recovery time was exceptionally difficult. She was not well-prepared mentally for the experience, nor was her Team, and this affected her overall attitude and motivation to make her own recovery easier. Since I had yet to go through surgery at that point, my advice was less effective. After knowing this, I expected my own recovery to be extremely difficult. By the end of week 6, when my bite-splint was removed, I almost felt like I had done something wrong because my recovery was relatively easy. The only exception is the anemia symptoms and that would not have been an issue if I had heeded the advice to refrain from exercising so soon.

- **Searching the internet for information on jaw surgery and recovery from blogs and videos is fine if you are also compiling a list of questions and concerns for your orthodontist and surgery appointments.** You NEED to communicate with your surgeon and with your orthodontist, and you NEED to make sure they are communicating with each other. For patients under 18, share the notebook with your parent(s) or guardian and encourage them to add questions and concerns of their own, and also to help you take notes during your appointments if they attend them with you. The better informed you are as a patient, the more compliant you will be with treatment. The more compliant you are with treatment, the better your results. It's a simple concept to understand, and a very simple concept to apply. Many patients who have used the Jaw Recovery Playbook for guidance throughout their surgery and recovery processes have found that keeping a notebook for questions, concerns, notes, and info was one of the most helpful things they did. It helped them remember information their surgeons said during appointments while they're in the midst of a mild panic attack after surgery worrying something was wrong when things were actually normal -- myself included!

- **Accept the fact that others will question whether jaw surgery is a good idea and no one but other jaw surgery patients will ever truly understand.** We are a special lot, jaw surgery patients, and we have suffered for most of our lives with conditions that many of us thought we simply had to live with. The dramatic change after jaw surgery can be more emotionally overwhelming than the entire process. As you grow accustomed to the changes, you will be so glad you had the opportunity to undergo corrective surgery AND you will be proud of yourself for managing your treatment and recovery with a positive attitude, quality nutrition, and diligent behavior. The extra effort it takes to heal well after jaw surgery is well worth it and the pride you will feel for doing so well will outshine almost any other experience in life.

- **Remember that this is a TEMPORARY SITUATION.** Compared to the rest of your life, jaw surgery treatment and recovery comprise only a fraction of your time. **Six weeks is a little over 11% of the year. If you live to be 75-years-old, the 6 weeks after jaw surgery will comprise roughly 0.15% of your lifetime; not even 1/4-percent. If you devote your attention and energy to improving your recovery experience through diligent nutrition, hydration, rest, and mental activity the time will pass very quickly and you will have an unbelievably EASY recovery.** You will be praised at every follow-up visit with your surgeon during those 6 weeks, and at your orthodontist's clinic as well. The praise feeds your motivation to continue working hard to heal WELL. It's worth it! Once it's over, it's over... with the exception of select patients who have more complicated initial cases requiring multiple surgeries or in the case of relapse, which is very rare for common procedures like ours.

- **Undergoing jaw surgery is NOT the same as breaking your jaw.** Countless patients choose specific wording when explaining to others that they will undergo jaw surgery. Saying that your surgeon will "break" your jaw sounds crude and barbaric. The wording will not help your attitude towards surgery and it may undermine efforts to remain positive. The concept of a broken jaw leaves many with the impression that you will be in extreme pain, disfigured, or worse, and that certainly doesn't improve non-patient impressions of why jaw surgery is "medically necessary" in cases such as ours. **Your surgeon went to**

school for a very long time to become skilled at oral & maxilofacial surgery procedures. They aren't pulling Residents out of class and sticking them in operating rooms, and you're not being physically operated on by unskilled or untrained providers. Surgeons with experience often state their experience somewhere in their office, business card, website, or informational brochures but if you're having surgery in a teaching hospital you should feel assured that your surgeon will likely be at least a fourth-year Resident assisted by another third- or fourth-year Resident, with a Staff Surgeon present to make sure things all go smoothly, plus some younger Residents may be present for observation.

- **The jaws are not broken but cut with extreme precision using specially designed tools for the absolute best possible outcome.** There are occasionally fractures that occur when the bones are cut or when the brackets and screws are applied after surgery which will often slow the recovery process slightly, but in no way, shape, or form is your surgeon creating a mess of your jaws so describing the surgery as a "break" or describing the jaw as "broken" is not only inaccurate, but it also undermines the level of skill involved in your surgeon's profession, as well as his or her training, efforts, experience, and professionalism. I find it offensive and insulting toward the surgeon when a patient takes this mindset. Surgery, by definition, involves careful planning, precise action, strategic focus, and skill.

> If that isn't convincing, remember that the surgeon will be adjusting your upper and/or lower jaw to correct a problem you were born with (or developed, such as after injury) and this is definitely a situation in which you want to be respectful, courteous, and considerate!

Understanding the Risks

When undergoing any type of surgery there are always risks involved. The benefits to the patient outweigh these risks, however, which is why surgery was offered as an option for you. Depending on the procedures selected for your case, the most common risk in jaw surgery patients is permanent nerve damage. The facial nerves are exposed during surgery and this exposure drives them nuts! Nerves are not meant to be seen, touched, or moved around so they shut down temporarily which results in a loss of sensation throughout the related areas of the face; usually the nose, cheeks, chin, lips, and often inside the mouth including gums and palate.

The degree to which the nerves go to sleep varies between patients, and the type of procedures undergone will influence which nerves are moved around. Some patients have some feeling back almost right away, or tingling such as the "pins & needles" sensation from Novocain when having cavities filled by a general dentist. Many patients experience some form of tingling sensation as the nerves wake up throughout recovery, and this can sometimes be perceived as painful especially if unaware of what's going on.

There are factors that affect the rate at which your body heals and the degree to which it heals. While many factors you can control, such as physical fitness, healthy bodyweight, proper sleep, staying hydrated, and eating well -- all of which I've discussed throughout this Playbook -- there are other factors you cannot control.

Age is a major factor in the way we heal. Patients undergoing jaw surgery who are in their teens and early 20s will heal significantly easier than patients in their 30s, 40s, or beyond. This does not mean that if you are in your 30s or 40s you cannot heal completely, but this should be understood for realistic expectation management.

The speed of healing will vary, especially with age. At 12 months, although most of the sensation returned to my face and mouth within the first 3 months after surgery, I still have tingling throughout my chin which can be sharp at times if I put significant pressure on my bottom lip (pressing up) or stretching the chin muscles in over-exaggerated movements. The sensation in my lower gums has returned fully but the upper gum-line is slightly dulled, as is my palate. It's not anything that I notice and it does not affect daily life or comfort; in fact, it may be a beneficial "loss" since some upper teeth were sensitive and they have since been less sensitive.

Some patients ask about relapse, but in my experience this is rarely a major problem. If you follow your surgeon's instructions throughout recovery, avoid chewing foods before you're given the okay to, and you adhere to your orthodontic treatment before and after surgery, including proper use of retainers after braces are removed, the possibility of relapse is significantly reduced. Even if you do not strictly use your retainers, the worst case scenarios is usually the teeth moving but your jaws will never be the way they were before surgery.

Research on Jaw Surgery Patients

A study of 170 patients before, throughout, and after orthognathic (corrective jaw) surgery was conducted in 2009 to evaluate the benefit of surgery to the quality of life of patients. A little over half the sample of patients were female (65%) and 40% of the patients underwent double-jaw surgery while 32% had upper-jaw surgery only.

Only 25% of these patients reported swelling perceived 3 weeks after surgery and less than 10% found the swelling a problem. By day 30, less than 3% of the patients had any perceived problem-swelling.

About 75% of these 170 patients reported no discomfort (or very slight discomfort) by day 18. By day 30, only 1-4% of the patients reported any pain or discomfort they felt was a problem.

Any problems with eating, chewing, opening the mouth, or talking were resolved within 6-8 weeks after surgery with over 75% of the patients with "chewing" taking the longest to return to "normal" -- but this is understandable since with most jaw surgeries the way the teeth come together is changed and we have to learn to properly chew, swallow, and speak with natural comfort.

Having undergone a period of speech therapy sessions in grade school with no emphasis on the eating aspects of tongue-thrust, I feared that I would need some form of treatment to learn to use the new jaw alignment properly. I consulted an SLP (speech-language pathologist) who, after assessing me completely, felt that I was really speaking and chewing properly but I was likely uncomfortable because I had to learn to find the new alignment "comfortable."

After 8 months post-surgery, I felt I was finally speaking, chewing, and swallowing naturally and with comfort. It takes time.

You may recall from the nutrition chapter how I recommend patients begin keeping track of their daily food and nutrition intake as well as daily activity or exercise. Research in jaw surgery patients conducted in 2008 showed that younger patients were more likely to keep track daily, when instructed to do so as part of a post-surgery protocol. My recommendations are made for all patients, regardless of age, because I know it will help. The daily food journal will show you that you are getting enough of what your body needs, but it will also allow you to see where you can improve. The daily exercise tracking will encourage you to stick to a routine and keep your body as healthy as possible. And when the surgery and recovery process is all over with you will be grateful to have this tangible record that you can look back on with pride.

TMJ Dysfunction Research

In 2010, research on TMJ dysfunction and orthognathic surgery was conducted involving 57 patients who underwent surgery between January 2006 and January 2008. The patients ranged in age from 16 to 65 and the 57 patients completed questionnaires regarding pain, sounds, clicking, joint locking, limited range of motion, and tension in their temporomandibular joints.

The questionnaire was sent to 176 patients, with only 57 responding, so keep that in mind the next time a hospital, doctor, or clinic requests your feedback. Those questionnaires can make a big difference in research that benefits many others.

The results of the study showed that most patients who experience some temporomandibular joint dysfunction before jaw surgery experienced improvement in TMJ-related symptoms and pain levels with corrective jaw surgery. Some patients without TMJ symptoms prior to surgery experienced the development of TMJ symptoms after surgery, but this was found to be an extremely low risk.

In my case, there were seven TMJ-related symptoms with orthodontic treatment in my teens, including locking open, during lunch usually, where I could not open or close any further until the jaw unlocked. There was also clicking, popping, and some aching, but it was never treated. Over time, the symptoms dissipated to only the occasional popping.

After surgery in 2011, there was considerable pressure on both TMJs during the first week post-surgery when I had so many bands holding my jaws shut that I could not part my teeth at all. I would yawn or cough a little and it would put significant pressure on the joints making me uncomfortable but it was more fear of damaging the jaws than pain. When the bands were removed, I had an almost grinding sound that was very noticeable whenever I would open my mouth wide or to express a full range of motion. This grinding wasn't painful but it was very loud to me. Over time, the grinding dissipated as well, and though it does occur at times, it is not painful and not as noticeable as it was.

When the surgeons corrected the way my jaws align they reduced unnecessary pressure on the TMJs which improved overall functioning and thus improved the symptoms I experienced in the past. Most patients experience improvement with TMJ issues, and research supports those claims.

Will you have the same experience? I can't promise you that. I can promise that it's realistically possible to see significant improvements in all your jaw-related issues with this type of corrective surgery.

6
What do I do if...?

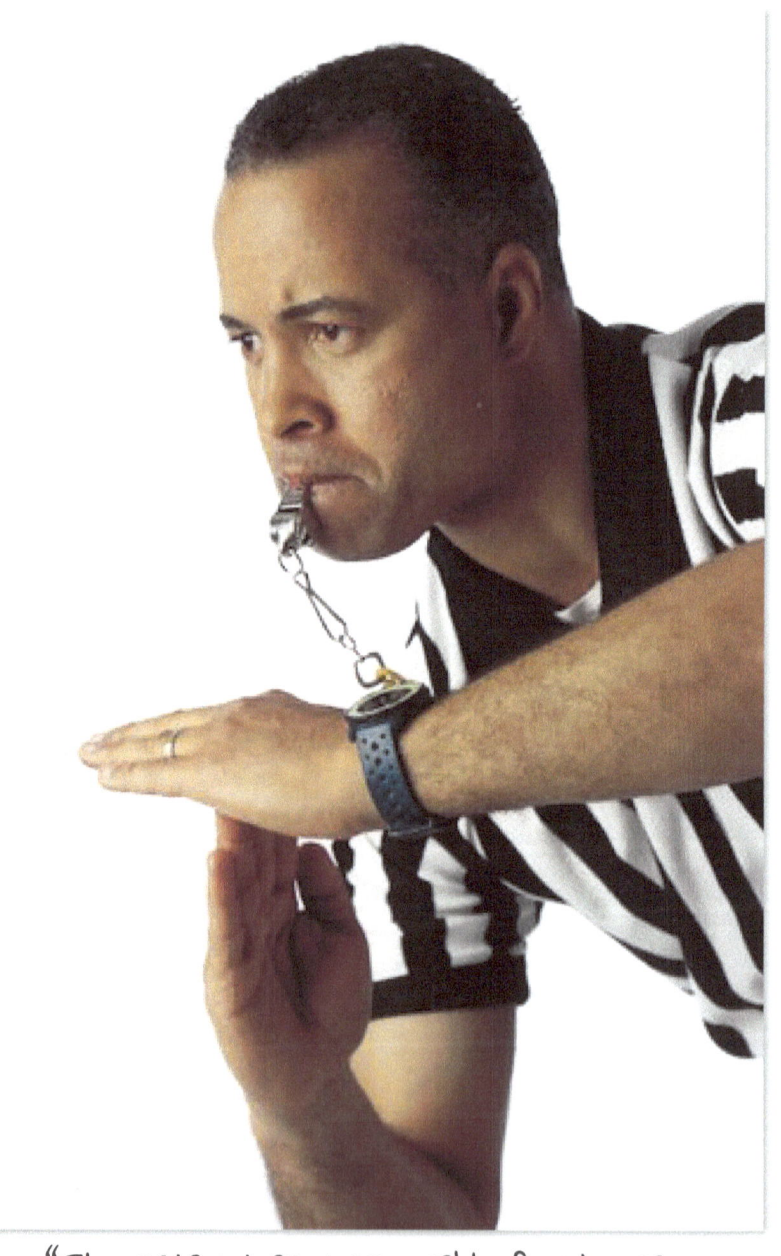

"The patient is responsible for keeping the different team components working together effectively." ~Sasha

My orthodontist said I'm ready BUT my surgeon said I'm not...

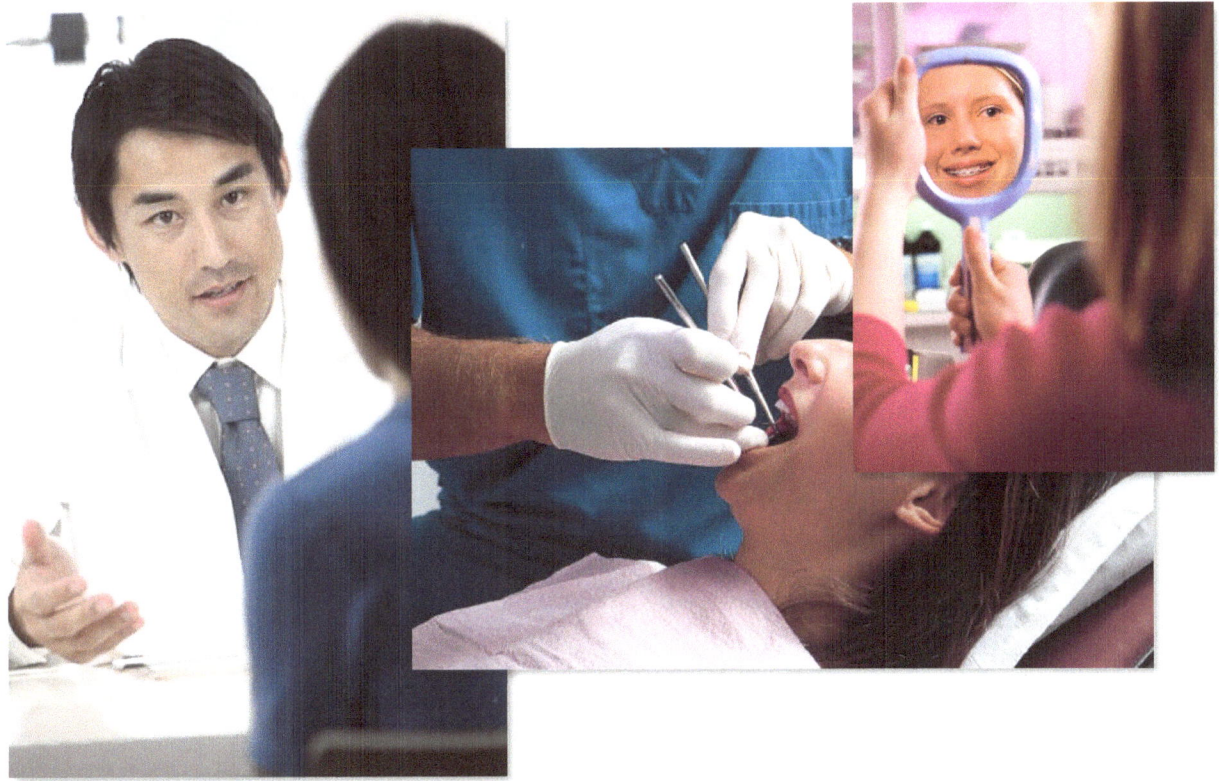

Several times throughout the Offense Playbook I mentioned being told by my orthodontist that I was ready for surgery only to be sent away by my surgeons who said I was not ready yet. This happened several times. Each time, as you can imagine, it was even more frustrating.

After about a year into my braces treatment, waiting for the surgery-ready "OK" from my surgeon, **I realized that the delays were ultimately my fault**. I hadn't been as proactive with the treatment process as I needed to be in order to speed things along.

I selected my orthodontist after researching the area I was living in. He is a civilian and among the top orthodontists in the area so I knew I couldn't go wrong.

I submitted his referral for jaw surgery to my general doctor at the time, and the referral was put into the computer at the military hospital. I assumed I would then make an appointment with a civilian surgeon, not realizing the military teaching hospital would treat me. I honestly didn't even know they offered oral & maxillofacial surgery. The referral was flagged by the teaching hospital and I was told I had to visit the OMFS clinic there first. If I wasn't happy with them I'd be able to find a civilian provider, if I wanted.

This was very convenient for me because then I didn't have to fight with my insurance company for coverage in a civilian hospital; by accepting treatment in the military hospital I would never see a bill. The problem, however, stemmed from the differences between military and civilian medical facilities. My surgeons communicate in typical military fashion, lacking a lot of the "fluff" to make sure the information is clearly understood. There is nothing wrong with that approach but between the limited communication and the changes every so-many months in my surgeon (from Residents moving around) I grew more frustrated when I realized my orthodontist was also feeling frustrated.

It took me a year to notice this because I only saw the OMFS staff a couple of times. Once I realized the communication short-coming I was able to clearly explain to the surgeons that they needed to be more clear and more direct with my orthodontist in order for him to do what they needed for my surgery.

It worked!

Don't Hesitate to HELP

Your surgeon and orthodontist NEED to communicate. My braces were on for about 6 months before I went to the surgeons again, under the impression I was nearly surgery-ready. I wasn't even close. I had to have brackets removed from my molars and bands put on them instead. I did that and went back when my orthodontist felt it was a good time again, about 8 months into my orthodontic treatment only to learn I then needed my wisdom teeth extracted and once they were extracted I would have to wait a minimum of 6 months before I could even be considered for surgery.

I went in for my wisdom teeth extraction, under the impression that all four were set to come out. Instead they removed only the bottom ones. This was done very quickly under local anesthesia (Novocain numbing my gums and nerves). I waited the 6 months and went back only to be told I still wasn't ready. That's about when I flipped out…

If I had known in advance that I was going to have to monitor and assist the communication lines between my providers, I would have been doing so from the very beginning and my treatment time might have been faster.

TALK to Your Orthodontist

Make sure your orthodontist is comfortable with the guidance provided by your surgeon. Make sure your orthodontist feels confident he understands what the surgeon wants in order to get you surgery-ready.

TALK to Your Surgeon

Surgeons are busy. You likely will have to leave messages and wait for calls when he's available. This is why having a notebook full of your questions and notes will improve the appointments with your surgeon. It'll save time because you won't have to remember (or risk forgetting) anything. When your surgeon calls back you'll be READY for a fast, efficient conversation.

No Matter What the Surgeon Says to YOU, He Should Contact the Orthodontist DIRECTLY to Relay Information Properly.

It is fine for you to take notes and ask the surgeon to explain exactly what he wants from the orthodontist, BUT do not take full responsibility for relaying this information. Tell your surgeon to please contact your orthodontist with the specific guidance regarding your future braces adjustments.

Arrive at your appointments PREPARED to give the surgeon the phone number to your orthodontist, even if you have given him the number several times in the past. This almost makes the surgeon seem unreliable but it's better to be diligent with your treatment management than to risk prolonging treatment needlessly by assuming they can handle it themselves. You're not their only patient.

This is YOUR treatment. The doctors may be friendly, but it matters little to them if you attend your appointments or not. It matters little to them if you ever get surgery-ready. They are really only concerned with your happiness with the end-results.

If you're hungry, are you going to wait for someone else to offer you food? No. That would be ridiculous.

If you are extremely thirsty, are you going to wait and see if someone offers you a drink of water? No. You're going to get it yourself.

Treat your surgery process with professional diligence by making sure you do what you have to do to get ready for surgery -- attend appointments, follow guidance from the orthodontist and surgeon, and follow the guidance in your Playbooks.

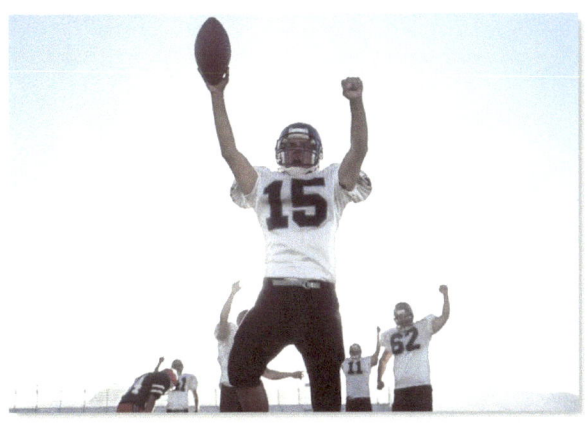

> Find order amongst the chaos and take control of your own jaw surgery process!
> ~ ~ ~ ~ ~
> TALK to your surgeon and orthodontist — encourage them to talk to each other for better, faster, and more efficient treatment planning.

Treat the members of your Team as if they are professionals paid to provide you with a service and you expect them to deliver. You don't have to harass the surgeon every day, but you're not his only patient so be prepared to contact him several times and make sure you speak with your orthodontist regularly to ensure he understands what the surgeon wants and expects. This will not only improve your overall treatment timeline but it will improve your satisfaction throughout the process.

It's YOUR treatment and surgery -- Manage it properly.

Be in control!

My Timeline Keeps Changing!

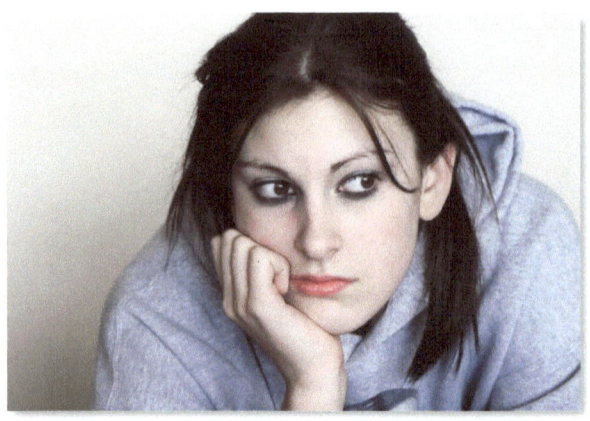

As soon as your braces are applied, it's difficult to refrain from expecting the timeline to remain constant. I am guilty of this too. As mentioned before, my initial surgeon predicted a 6-8 month timeline before I'd be surgery-ready, then about 3-4 months after surgery and recovery he predicted my braces would come off. In reality my upper and lower jaws were not ready for surgery until over 14 months after the braces were applied, and it was still another two months before I was in the operating room. But it wasn't simply a "you're just not ready" situation. Three times my orthodontist felt I was ready, according to the guidance provided by the surgical team, and three times they sent me back to my orthodontist with completely new instructions.

> It should be noted that in 100% of the jaw surgery patients I have worked with over the past three years, every patient was given one prediction before their braces were put on, and every patient had to wait longer than the predicted timeline before they were ready for surgery.

I had my braces applied in the first week of July 2010. In November I went in for an appointment with my surgical team to assess my progress; that would be my second appointment with them. I wanted an update before the New Year.

At that appointment, I spent several hours between having impressions made, photos taken, X-rays, measurements, and talking with the surgeons and Residents. I then waited two weeks for a decision and learned that I wasn't ready, but also my braces needed some changes in order for me to prepare for surgery. While it's not true for all patients, many surgeons prefer metal bands around the molars to prevent trouble if brackets are knocked loose during the procedures. I didn't have these bands to start with so at my next orthodontist appointment bands were placed over eight molars. Not very comfortable, but a necessary "evil" in my case.

I returned for my second follow-up with the surgeons a few months later, to see if I was closer to being surgery-ready. I was informed then, that I needed my wisdom teeth extracted. I was also informed that once the wisdom teeth were pulled, I would have to wait at least 6 months before surgery would even be an option because the jaw needed to heal from the extractions. You can imagine how thrilled I was to hear this…

I couldn't get an appointment for the extractions for over a month, and when I went for the extractions they decided only to take the bottom wisdom teeth that time. I insisted that if the top teeth also needed extraction, they should take them all to save me the trouble of an additional 6-month wait but they assured me that if the top wisdom teeth needed to be out they could simply "pop" them out during surgery.

The lower wisdom teeth were extracted by the Resident that became my third and final jaw surgeon. He was able to take both lower wisdom teeth in only a matter of minutes! I chose to have local anesthesia only, rather than be knocked out for such a simple procedure. I was surprised at how well the Novocain worked because I typically have trouble with it for fillings. It took about 25 minutes to prepare me for the extraction and he was done, both teeth out, in only a few minutes so it wasn't bad at all.

I returned 6 months later for another screening and was told I still wasn't ready. It was around this time that I learned what a teaching hospital is and it was around this time that I finally snapped into "business" mode and made sure that my surgeon and orthodontist were talking. I was very upset when I went in after so long and so many changes, only to be told a third time that I still wasn't ready. I just about bit my surgeon's head off with my snappy attitude and that wasn't really fair to him because he hadn't been my surgeon the whole time. It certainly didn't make me feel any better. But it worked. He took the time to call and talk with my orthodontist himself, clearly explaining exactly what they needed done, and at my next orthodontic appointment my orthodontist explained to me what was really going on.

He explained why the surgeon had been changed three times, that the hospital is a teaching hospital, what that means, and he explained what they needed before I'd be ready for surgery.

After that appointment, I made the choice to change my attitude. I apologized for snapping at him when I saw my surgeon again, and at every subsequent appointment I was considerably more patient and considerably more sociable than I had been previously.

Taking an attitude to those appointments wasn't going to make the 2-3 hours go any faster. It wasn't going to make them any more willing to help me faster. It wasn't going to make me feel any better, and it certainly wasn't going to make them want to help me. **I didn't want to be THAT patient, so I changed.**

After surgery there were also a significant amount of changes to the timeline that would have left me frustrated if I didn't continue this attitude. For example, my orthodontist explained that most patients that undergo surgery have their braces off within a few months. I allowed this to become an expectation which led to a little disappointment for myself. That's my fault...poor expectation management when it came to the completion of my braces.

It took 13 months (and a day) after surgery for my braces to finally come off. There were issues closing gaps between teeth. Surprisingly, not the teeth where the surgery gaps were made. Ultimately, my orthodontist had to use a tiny file to smooth the inner sides of some teeth, allowing them to fit nicer. Teeth aren't rectangles. If they were, they'd line up easier. Instead, they're more like triangles. This was creating gaps near the gum line between certain teeth but they wouldn't move any closer because the lower portions were close together.

My first premolars on the bottom were also a little problematic. The premolars are bicuspids, meaning the teeth contain two cusps or bump-like ridges on the top. My upper bicuspids are true bicuspids with both cusps present and accounted for, resembling two little mountains. With my lower bicuspids, however, the first premolars are single-cusp teeth. They're missing the lingual cusp (the one on the inside of the tooth near my tongue). This made them stubborn to turn into position and stubborn to line up right with the surrounding teeth.

I joked with my orthodontist that since the lingual cusp is "non-functional" it's actually not missing. It's a sign that I'm just more evolved since my genes recognized its uselessness and didn't code for the lingual cusps to grow. In reality, it's just luck of the draw, I think, and not actually as awesome as being more evolved. (There goes my chance to join the X-Men…)

So what does this mean for you and your case?

It could mean nothing. My situation is not the standard; it's an example. Your orthodontist and surgeon may provide a guess at a timeline that proves true. They could provide a predicted timeline of 12 months to surgery and you might not be surgery-ready for 24 months.

The choices you make during your treatment as preparation for surgery can influence your timeline. If your teeth are healthy and move at a normal pace, your timeline might be shorter than the prediction. If you frequently miss appointments with your orthodontist, don't use bands as instructed, eat foods and candy you're told to avoid, and generally don't take control of the situation (regardless of your age), your timeline could double or triple.

Basically, if you want your treatment to be as quick as possible, you have to take the time and make the effort to work with your providers to improve your speed and overall results. But you also must maintain a sense of "expectation management" so you are not completely thrown off balance when things change, and then change again. You could do everything perfectly and still be delayed by six months or a year or longer simply because you opted for the cheapest braces or even if you chose the self-ligating braces, as I did, you could still be delayed by nature; if your teeth are stubborn or there's an unforeseen problem that slows the orthodontics process, there's nothing you can do. Accept it, and do the best you can to stay the course with a good attitude.

I mentioned "regardless of age" because several patients among the hundreds I've worked with have been teenagers. Teenage patients typically feel that the parents are responsible for their treatment and while that's technically legally the case, **the patient is ALWAYS -- ALWAYS -- ALWAYS the Quarterback.** As the patient, you are ALWAYS in control, even if you don't see it. There is nothing stopping you from asking your surgeon "Did you speak to my orthodontist on the phone?" And there is nothing stopping your from asking your orthodontist, "Did you speak with my surgeon on the phone?"

Ask them if they both understand what's going on. If your orthodontist seems frustrated or unsure, tell your surgeon he or she needs to contact them and verify that everything is going smoothly.

Don't be lazy. Don't let the grown-ups mess things up. It's easy to get lost in the grown-up world of professional fields and it's easy for grown-ups to get confused when they're not communicating effectively.

You want your treatment to be as concise as possible so you have the best results possible. The only way to ensure this is to force the people involved to keep communicating.

They will appreciate the initiative, if you take it.

I'm sick of this!

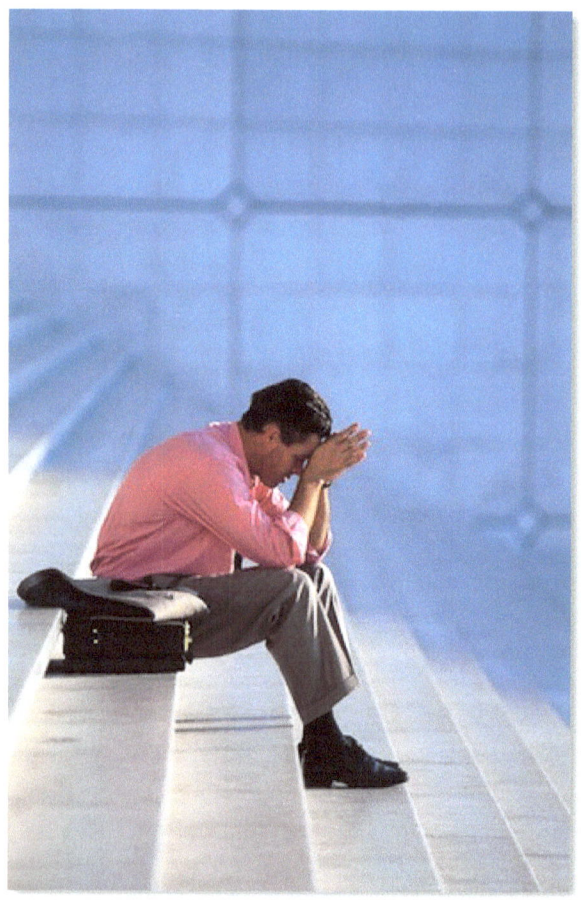

We all get this way at times, especially when things keep changing and we feel we have no control. While it's especially true of younger patients who feel the parents and doctors are in control of their fate, adult patients also feel frustrated because as adults we expect to be able to make choices and control things yet with jaw surgery we're faced with a lot of waiting, a lot of changes, and sometimes insufficient or inefficient communication between the providers, but also between the providers and ourselves. We're facing a lot of "unknowns" and it's scary. We have everyday life still stressing us out, and we're uncomfortable from regular orthodontic treatment. We just want it over with and we want it over with YESTERDAY!

I know. I've been there too.

While nothing I say will make the frustration and stress disappear, there are ways you can control how much these things affect you. If you focus on the day-by-day process, the little details of every bit of your treatment while you work up to being surgery-ready, the time is going to drag on and seem never-ending.

It helps to remember the reason you sought jaw surgery and treatment in the first place. How uncomfortable it was to smile so you often avoided pictures. How uncomfortable it was to eat, especially in public, so you'd avoid eating out with friends or you'd always feel stuck ordering something you knew you could eat neatly without much trouble. How uncomfortable it was to speak because the malocclusion or other issue caused speech difficulties, such as the lisp I grew up fighting.

Jaw surgery is a wonderful gift. An expensive gift, mind you, but a wonderful gift for yourself. **It's the chance to completely change the way you feel about your appearance, your speech, your chewing and swallowing habits, and your overall comfort with your mouth.** Although every patient has a different circumstance and these issues may not always apply, **I am 100% certain that you have a list of your own, regarding all the struggles that brought you to this decision for jaw surgery.**

Hold on to that list. Don't lose sight of the difficulties and don't, for even a moment, try to think that perhaps things weren't that bad or perhaps you could live with the issues.

It's very easy to second-guess our decisions when the process to reach the end result is a long one. **If those struggles were something you were willing to live with, you never would have considered jaw surgery.** *Remember that!* By improving your occlusion, no matter what the starting problem was, you are improving your long-term quality of life which will make you happier and healthier. **Jaw surgery will help you do that by giving you the alignment and functional structure your body was meant to have. It's worth it.**

Even if you can't see it now, you will soon be able to look back on the way you felt throughout your surgery preparations and you'll be so glad that you stuck it out. Glad that you took charge and made your Team the best it could possibly be for your treatment and recovery. So glad that you went through with it, despite the struggles and frustration. *You might be so glad that you'll send your story to the Jaw Recovery Playbook to help inspire other patients who are in that same boat now!*

7

Jaw Recovery Playbook

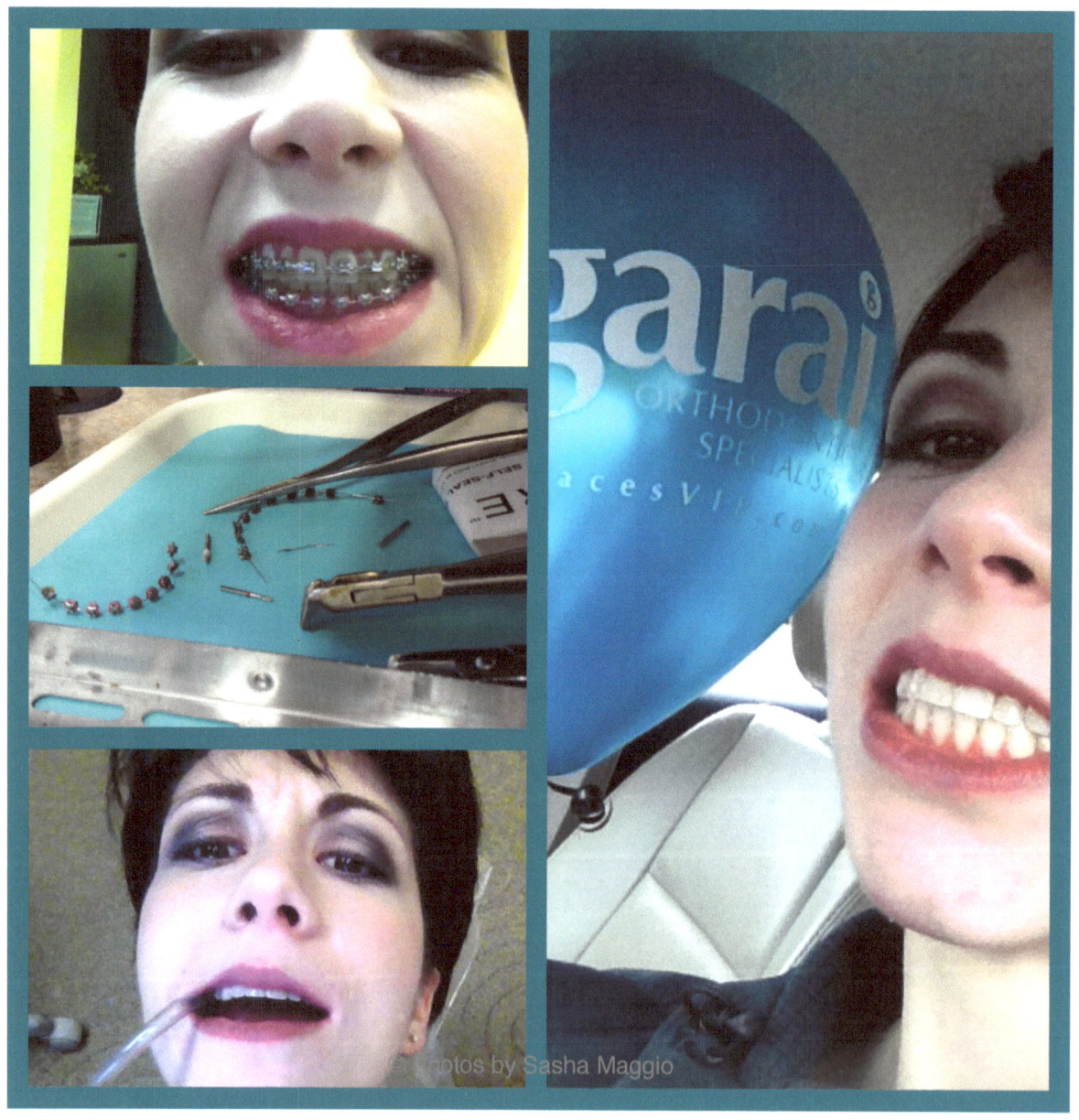

"Jaw surgery is SO WORTH IT!"
~ Sasha

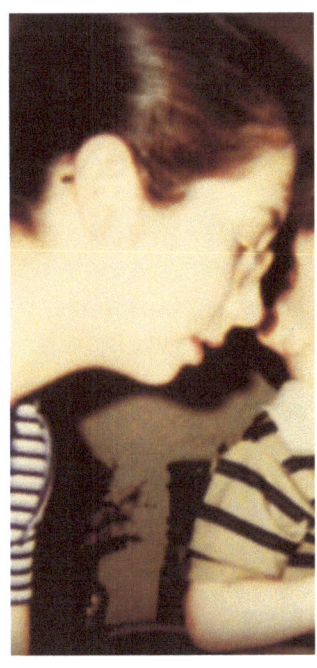
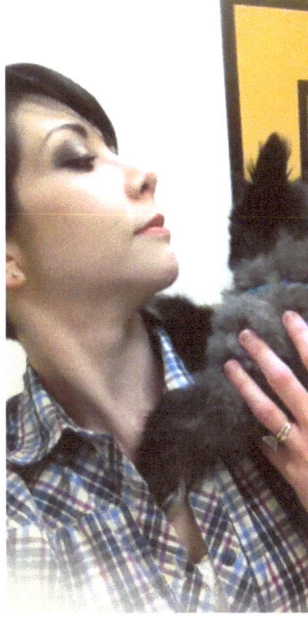

(left) 1999 to 2000-ish
(right) April 2013

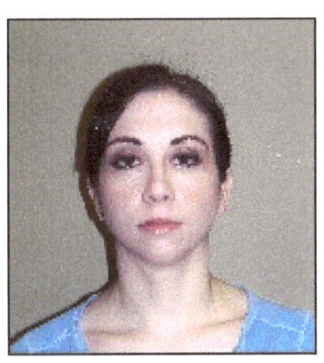

June 2010, taken at Garai Orthodontics before braces were put on the following month.

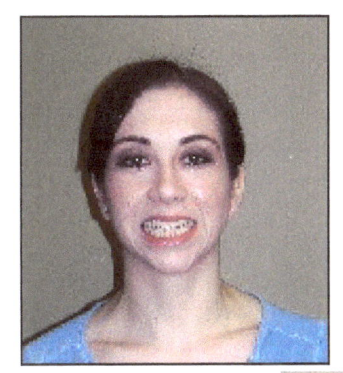

Passport photos, taken in April 2013
The first set I did at a drugstore and seriously cried because they were so awful. A very sweet photographer that worked in the hospital's Med Photo Lab offered to retake them for me and they were so much better I cried again!

© Photos by Sasha Maggio

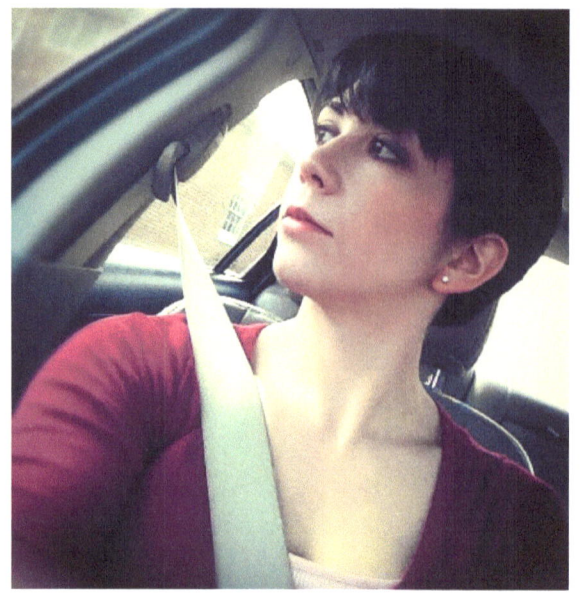

It took me longer to adjust to the subtle changes than I anticipated. I had revision surgery in March 2013 to repair my nose (I had an issue breathing from the way things healed) and the remove the hardware from the first surgery. It is not always removed, in fact it rarely is in the U.S. but it was causing some muscle-pulling that affected my comfort to such a degree that removing it was worth the added risk of a second surgery.

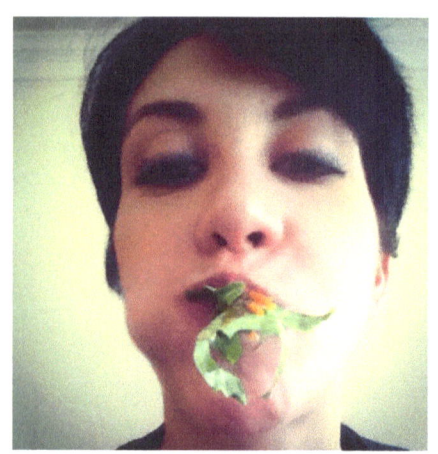

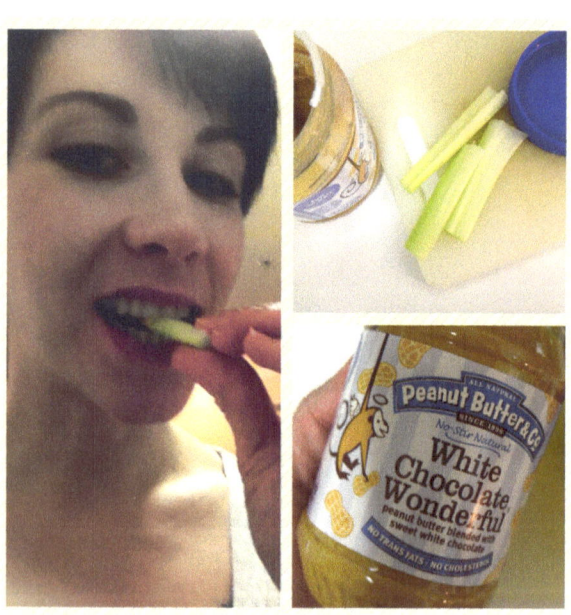

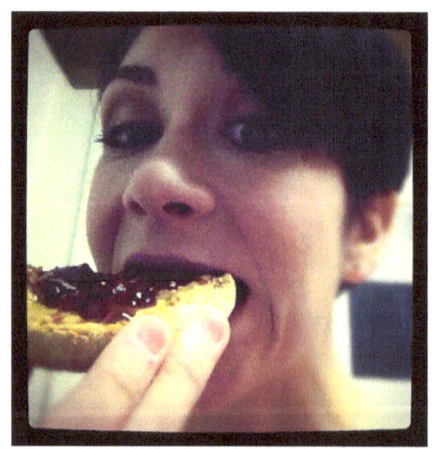

I never thought I'd enjoy chewing so much — EVER!

© Photos by Sasha Maggio

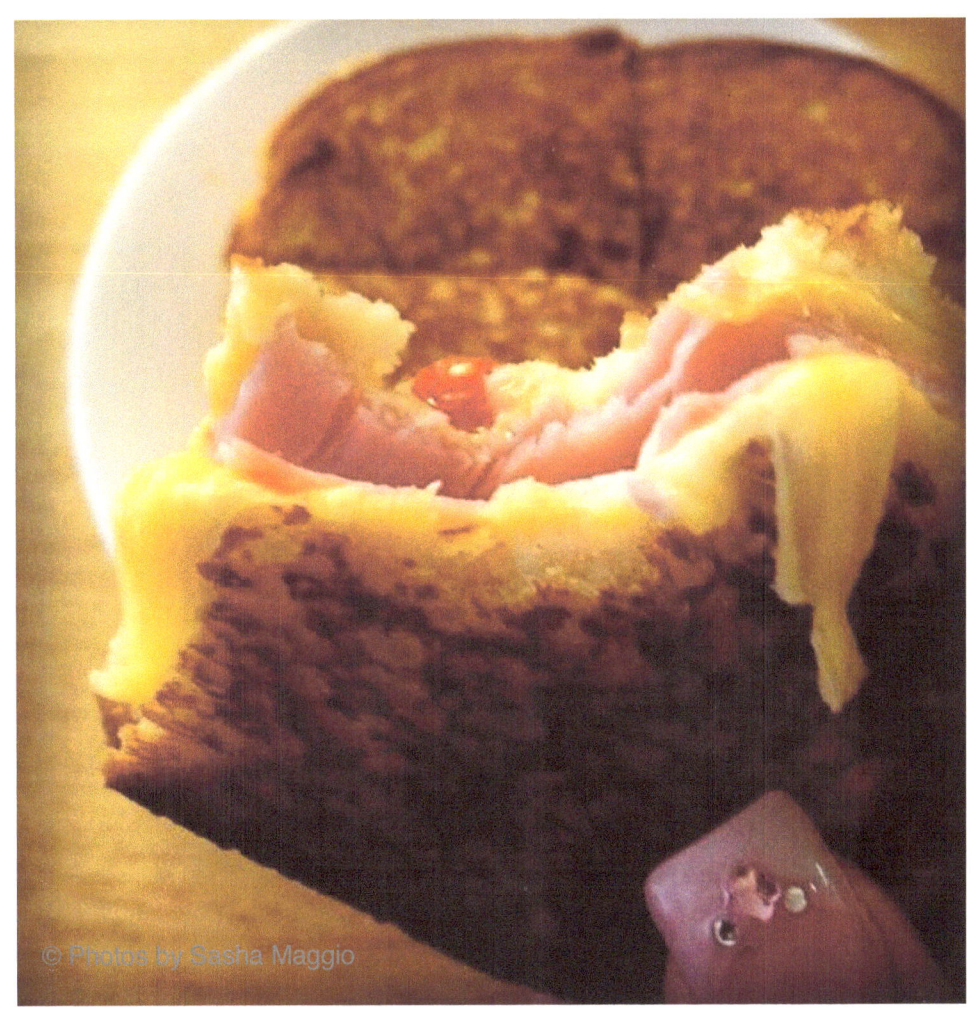

The very first time I used my front teeth to bite into something….

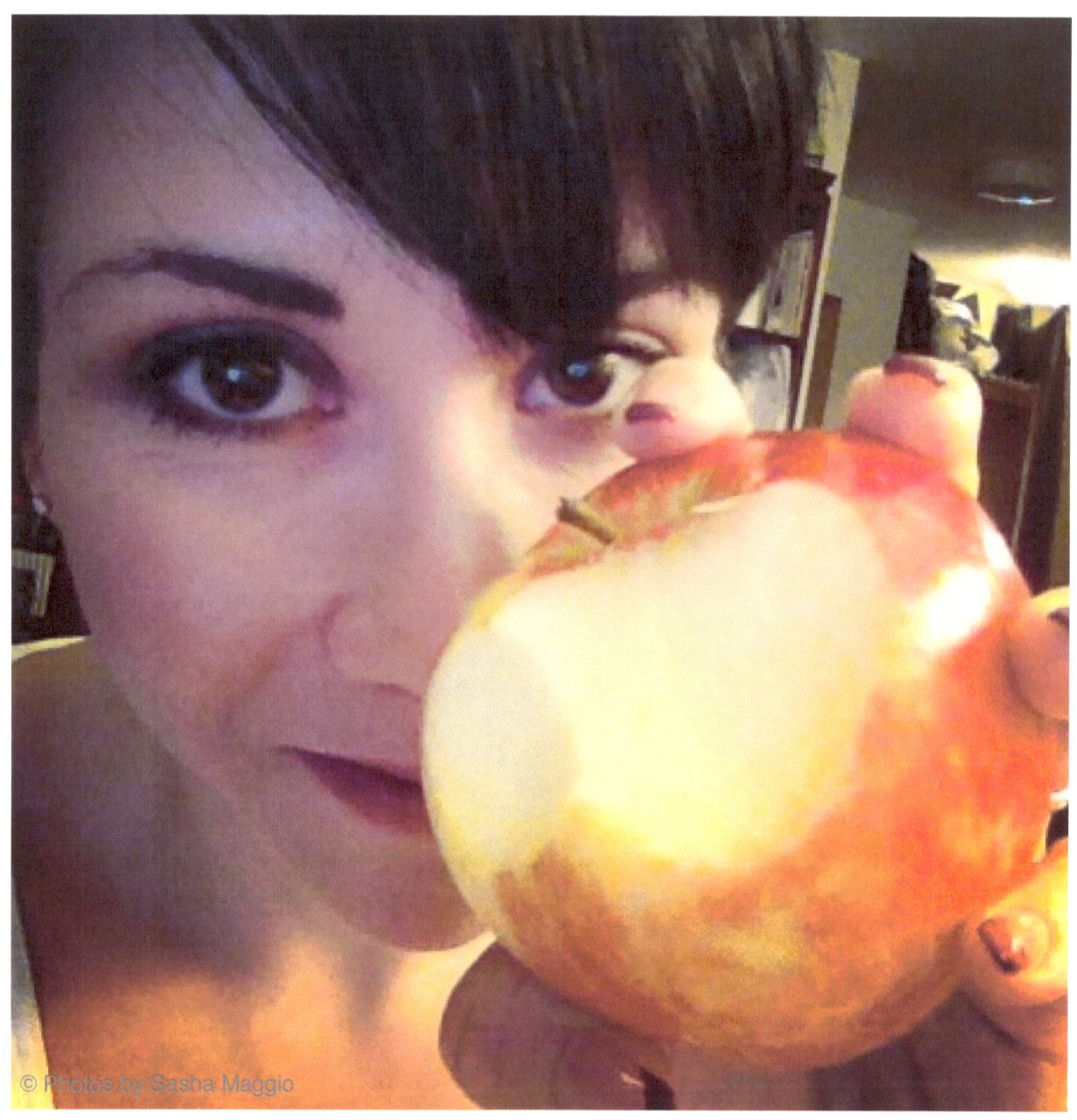

First time using my front teeth to bite into an apple! January 2014 — Even after my braces were off I kept cutting them up. I went to grab a knife and then stopped myself and thought "No, you put time, effort, and money into this bite, you should use it!"

I created the Jaw Recovery Playbook as a way to share the ~~hundreds~~ thousands of hours of research I had conducted for my own surgery and recovery. I could not, in good conscience, keep that work to myself because so much effort went into it and it made my recovery so much easier. How could I sleep at night knowing other patients didn't even know where to begin?

It took a long time to get organized, though. Between post-surgery anemia and another health issue, full-time work, managing student loans (ha!) and preparing for another military move -- balancing time became the struggle.

While every patient has a different experience with their surgery and recovery, most patients that have contacted me through the Jaw Recovery Playbook have reported having an easier recovery, an easier time maintaining a positive attitude throughout even the difficult days, faster swelling reduction after surgery, better diet after surgery, and generally a surprisingly fast recovery pace.

The ~~dozens~~ hundreds of patients I've helped since my own surgery has increased to over a hundred! The replies and feedback I've received from these patients has kept me motivated to continue working through the research and notes and finally organizing the **Jaw Recovery Playbook SYSTEM**, which I've designed to help all members of the surgery team. The patient, the family and friends involved in the patient's recovery, the surgeons and orthodontists - Every member has a Playbook designed to help THEM in an effort to improve the patient's surgery and recovery experience.

The Recipe Playbook began at just under 100 pages; full of recipes I used during my own initial 6-week recovery, and now has expanded to include even more nutrition information and even more recipes — nearly double the original Playbook!

The Game Day & Recovery Playbook walks the patient and team through the pre-surgery appointment, the surgery process, waking up in the hospital after surgery, and the first 6 weeks of recovery, while also offering helpful tips and suggestions for improving the overall pace at which the patient recovers.

How you use the Jaw Recovery Playbook System is up to you. Some patients simply want the basic info and recipes, while other patients want all the details and obsessively prepare for all they can -- like I did. It is my hope that the System I created can serve as a blueprint for helping as many jaw surgery patients as possible, with a flexibility that allows the patient to understand how some things are different while most things are the same for all of us.

Visit the Jaw Recovery Playbook for access to a variety of resources and please feel free to submit photos, stories, and testimonials to help improve the Jaw Recovery Playbook System so that it can help even more jaw surgery patients!

Share the website with your family and friends, who will become your support team during your surgery and recovery process, and with your orthodontist and surgeons.

They may be interested in the Offensive Coordinator Playbook, designed specifically for orthodontists and surgeons to improve patient understanding and satisfaction. Great care was taken to create a Playbook just for the providers because I feel that improving their communication efforts and understanding of jaw surgery patients will dramatically improve overall patient satisfaction in almost any case.

Thank you for trusting the Jaw Recovery Playbook to help you through your jaw surgery experience!

8
Where do I go next?

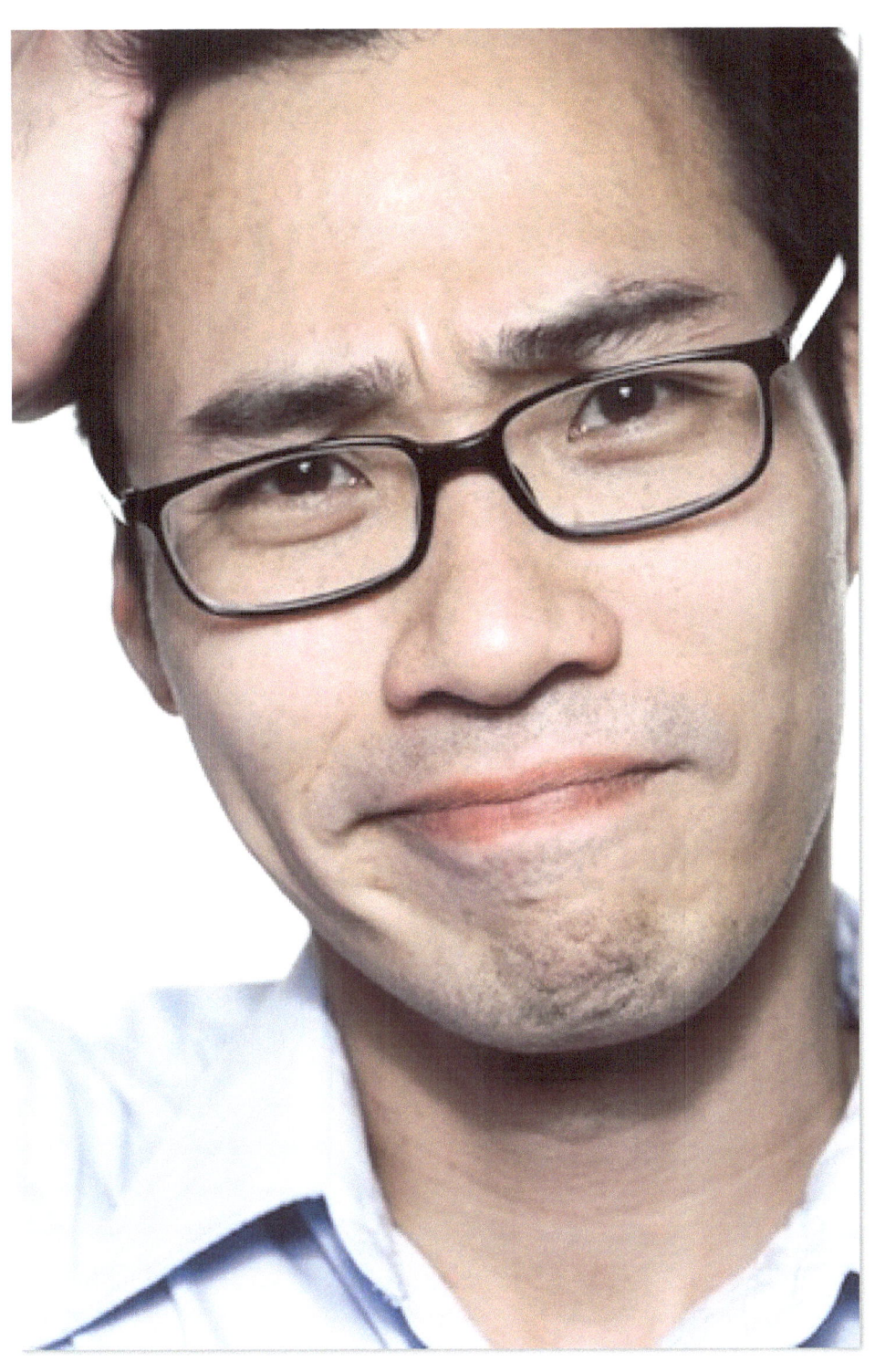

Thank you for reading the Jaw Recovery Playbook Offense Playbook! You should now feel more comfortable about the path ahead, to braces, surgery, recovery, and beyond. The Offense Playbook is designed to help patients gain a better understanding of their circumstances and what they can do now to prepare for surgery later. The Defense Playbook is similar, but designed to help the patient's family or support team with that process.

The Game Day & Recovery Playbook combines two very important aspects of your jaw surgery experience. The first part of the playbook will walk you through the process of setting up your appointment for surgery, once your surgeon has determined you are ready, then the pre-surgery appointment and the day of surgery. This part of the Game Day & Recovery Playbook will help you know what to expect, what the experience is like, and how you can prepare for it. The second part of the playbook addresses the initial 6 weeks of your recovery after surgery. This includes managing your medication, knowing when something is wrong and when something odd is actually normal, maximizing your time to improve recovery efforts, and steps you can take to speed up recovery (within reason).

The Recipe Playbook contains the same recipes I developed during my recovery, with nutrition information and additional nutrition guidance. Since recovering from surgery I have DOUBLED the recipe content so you will have plenty of variety with both sweet and savory options to please any palate.

The Braces Playbook is designed for both jaw surgery patients and non-jaw surgery patients. This playbook explains the process of orthodontic treatment in a general sense, along with guidance for managing your self-care and oral hygiene throughout the treatment. There are plenty of tips and recommendations to help any patient with braces, whether having surgery or not. For patients with braces but not having surgery, the Recipe Playbook also makes a great companion to your Braces Playbook for when your teeth are sore after an adjustment!

The Offensive Coordinator Playbook is not really for patients, but instead offers suggestions and insight for Oral & Maxillofacial Surgeons (and related professionals) to help the providers help their patients more efficiently. There are sections that address the surgery experience from the patient-side, as well as patient psychology and communication strategies for building CONFIDENCE, not just rapport. Patients are welcome to purchase the Offensive Coordinator Playbook if they wish, and I encourage patients to recommend the Offensive Coordinator Playbook and the Jaw Recovery Playbook System to their orthodontist and surgeon. A lot of effort was put into this System to help improve patient compliance and patient satisfaction, which can benefit the providers as well.

Lastly, the Jaw Recovery Playbook website, www.JawRecoveryPlaybook.com, offers free resources and sample chapters of the six Playbooks, videos, presentations, and options for even more support.

This is YOUR surgery experience. YOU have control over how easy or how difficult the different stages are for you, and your choices will affect your TEAM, your orthodontist, and your surgeon. Let's work together to make this an enjoyable experience for everyone!

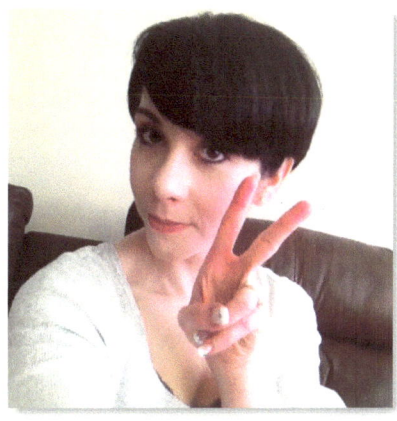

~Sasha

Glossary

About this Glossary Chapter...

The integrated Glossary function for iBooks does not display completely on PDF versions of this Playbook so I have changed from using the interactive glossary to using this Glossary Chapter for universal convenience. The Glossary contains words that some patients may already know, while many do not. It is simply to enhance comprehension when preparing for jaw surgery or managing orthodontic and surgery treatment. Many of the words may appear in bold throughout the Playbook text, which denotes their link to the integrated glossary entry for that particular word.

~Sasha

> communication is key!
> If you do not understand your surgeon when he speaks to you, ASk for clarification. If you think your orthodontist is unclear on something, make sure he is communicating with your surgeon to improve your treatment and care!

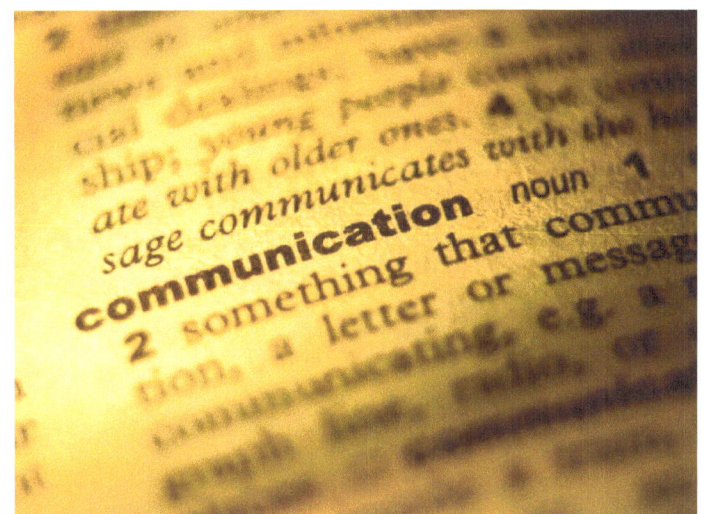

Alignment: The way your teeth come together when you close your upper and lower jaws.

~~~~~~~~~~

Archwires: The horizontal wire that runs through the brackets on your teeth. This wire is held in place by small ties placed over each bracket; in the past the ties were individual wires twisted and clipped with the ends tucked behind the archwire. On self-ligating braces the archwire is held in place by latches on each bracket.

~~~~~~~~~~

Bilateral Sagittal Split Osteotomy: A surgical procedure in which the lower jaw is cut (osteotomy) inward, at both sides (bilateral), then the cut is angled to create a wedge-style slice (sagittal split) at the sides of the mandible (lower jaw). The front portion of the lower jaw is then moved and secured for a proper alignment.

This procedure involves moving the front portion of the lower jaw, containing the bottom teeth, and often adjusts the patient's profile for a more-desirable appearance as an added benefit to the functional improvements.
Also referred to as a **BSSO.**

~~~~~~~~~~

Bite: The contact between top teeth and bottom teeth when the mouth is closed and the upper jaw and lower jaw are brought together.

~~~~~~~~~~

BSSO: Bilateral Sagittal Split-Osteotomy

~~~~~~~~~~

Corrective Surgery: An operation performed with the goal of improving a physical or physiological problem. In corrective jaw surgery, the upper jaw, lower jaw, or both jaws are adjusted for improved functioning, alignment, and appearance.

Although corrective surgery can have cosmetic benefits, the goal of the surgery is first to improve functionality. This is why corrective jaw surgery is able to be labeled as "medically necessary" and covered by many health insurance providers.

~~~~~~~~~~

Cosmetic Surgery: A surgical procedure performed solely for aesthetic purposes. Unlike corrective surgery, which contains a medically necessary aspect, cosmetic surgery may be performed simply to improve the patient's appearance.

Cosmetic surgery is also known as plastic surgery, aesthetic plastic surgery, or medical aesthetics.

Common cosmetic surgery procedures include genioplasty (chin surgery), rhinoplasty (nose job), and lip enhancements. Corrective jaw surgery is a medically necessary procedure for the majority of patients but it does often include improved appearance for a secondary cosmetic benefit.

~~~~~~~~~~

Defense: The Defense traditionally works to combat an opposing team's offense, but in the Jaw Recovery Playbook the "Defense" is composed of the patient's support team. The support team will often consist of one or more parents, siblings, and other family members, particularly in the case of younger patients. Older patients' teams may contain a spouse or partner, children, or extended family.

In football, this support team is more like the Offensive Line, but to keep the theme balanced I opted to make the support team the patient's Defensive Line.

~~~~~~~~~~

Game Day: Game Day refers to the date of the surgery. In the Game Day Playbook you will find information to help you prepare for your Game Day and your brief hospital stay. The Recovery Playbook covers your 6-12 week recovery period.

~~~~~~~~~~

General Dentist: The General Dentist is a dentistry professional, usually DMD or DDS, that specializes in preventative care and repair of teeth. You visit your general dentist for annual or biannual cleanings and check-ups, and your general dentist will drill & fill cavities, repair fillings, and often perform root canals and crowning procedures.

Cosmetic dentistry, such as bleaching, whitening, porcelain veneers, dentures, bridges, and related services are sometimes performed by general dentists as part of regularly available services in a particular clinic.

~~~~~~~~~~

General Doctor: You General Doctor is one who you visit for annual physical exams, common health problems, and minor injuries or illnesses. As opposed to a specialist, the general doctor manages your everyday health through regular check-ups and treatment as needed.

A general doctor may be an MD or OD. Also referred to as a **PCM** (primary care manager) or **PCP** (primary care physician), in some healthcare facilities.

~~~~~~~~~~

Genioplasty: Chin surgery, often including augmentation or reduction. A chin implant may be used or the front portion of the lower jaw may be cut and repositioned for improved appearance. Bone graft may be used for better healing and titanium brackets and screws generally comprise the assembly for non-magnetic lasting support.

Genioplasty is a cosmetic procedure but often found in conjunction with corrective jaw surgery procedures to improve the patient's overall satisfaction after healing.

~~~~~~~~~~

Invisalign: An alternative to traditional braces, Invisalign is an orthodontic treatment that uses clear teeth aligners to gently move teeth for improved appearance and functionality.

Invisalign is generally not an option for jaw surgery patients because the surgeon will need brackets on the front surfaces of the teeth with archwires and surgical hooks in order to perform the surgery. Although more expensive, a patient may opt for Invisalign throughout the initial preparation and after recovery from jaw surgery provided the patient has standard braces at the time of surgery. This option, however, will depend on the procedures and preparations needed.

www.invisalign.com

~~~~~~~~~~

Jaw Recovery Playbook: The Jaw Recovery Playbook is a comprehensive resource for jaw surgery patients, orthodontists, oral & maxilofacial surgeons and residents, and caregivers helping jaw surgery patients through their surgery and recovery. It was designed by Sasha Maggio, a jaw surgery patient, after hundreds of hours of scientific, scholarly, and social research into jaw surgery, recovery, healing, nutrition, and health.

The Jaw Recovery Playbook includes a variety of individual Playbooks which serve as guides for the patient, the orthodontist and surgeons, the patient's family or caregivers, and others involved.

www.JawRecoveryPlaybook.com

~~~~~~~~~~

Jaw Surgery: Also referred to as oral surgery, oral & maxillofacial surgery, orthognathic surgery, and corrective jaw surgery, jaw surgery is any surgical procedure involving the mouth including the teeth, jaw bones, and temperomandibular joints.

~~~~~~~~~~

Le Fort I: Le Fort fractures refer to skull fractures or cuts involving the upper jaw or maxillary bone. There are three levels for the Le Fort fractures, with Le Fort I the most common among jaw surgery patients. It is technically referred to as an "osteotomy" (bone surgery) but I refer to it as a "procedure" in most places for simplicity.

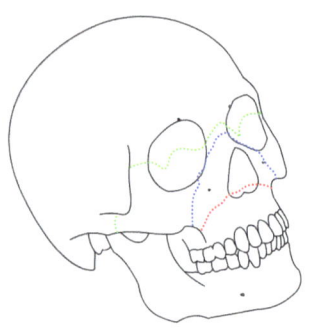

The Le Fort I osteotomy is the cut surgeons make which runs above the roots (apices) of the upper teeth through the nasal septum to the lateral pyriform rims. The Le Fort I cut is below the zygomaticomaxillary junction (where the cheek bones meet the upper jaw bone) and interrupts the pterygoid plates (near the back of the palate forming part of the boundary of the nasal cavity) by way of the pterygomaxillary junction. This is a lot of big, scary words that intimidate many jaw surgery patients -- try to remember that they are just words!

This can sound confusing and scary to those without a solid understanding of cranial anatomy - to simplify, try this exercise:

- Stand in front of a mirror with full view of your face.
- Take your two pinkie fingertips and place one on each side of your nose.
- With your index fingers, feel for your cheek bones and place one index finger on each cheek bone to mark their location.
- Now take your middle finger and ring finger tips and position them on your lower cheek, lower than the cheek bones and slightly angled downward from where your pinkies are next to your nose.
- The line that would connect the six (middle, ring, and little) fingers is the approximate location of your Le Fort I cut line. This will vary, but it gives a general idea for comprehension. The red line in the skull is the Le Fort I mark.

Common symptoms of a cut (surgical) or fracture (injury) at the Le Fort I level include swelling of the upper lip and cheeks, and bruising along the cheeks.

In the event of a Le Fort I fracture from injury, the upper teeth may become loose and the teeth alignment (occlusion) may be affected -- but these are avoided in surgery by careful planning and surgical bone cuts above the teeth apices (roots).

~~~~~~~~~~

Lingual Braces: Lingual braces are brackets designed to attach to the lingual side of the teeth; the side that faces the tongue. The goal of lingual braces is to hide their presence but they will not be suitable for most jaw surgery patients do to the surgical needs for brackets and archwires on the front surface of teeth.

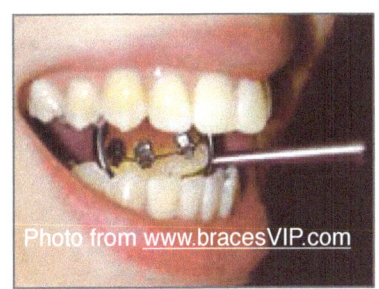

For general information about where to find Lingual Braces in your area visit the American Lingual Orthodontics Association at www.lingualbraces.org

~~~~~~~~~~

Macronutrients: Nutrients needed in large quantities by the body. Macronutrients are measured in grams and include protein, carbohydrates, and lipids. Water is usually grouped with macronutrients, as well.

~~~~~~~~~~

Malocclusion: A misalignment of the teeth or some relevant difference between the upper teeth and lower teeth that affects the way they come together and function.

Occlusion refers to the alignment of the teeth; mal- is a (French, Latin-based) prefix meaning "illness" or "bad"

~~~~~~~~~~

Mandible: The lower jaw. The mandible is also referred to as the inferior maxillary bone. It holds the bottom teeth and forms the shape of the jawline and chin.

The temperomandibular joint or TMJ is a common source of pain, clicking, and locking problems for people with poor alignment of the upper and lower jaws.

~~~~~~~~~~

Maxilla: The maxilla is composed of two upper jaw bones (the maxillae), connecting at the midline (center of the face). The maxilla helps house the upper teeth and helps form the palate (roof of the mouth), as well as helping form the nasal antrum and the eye orbits.

The tops of the maxillae border the zygomatic bones (cheek bones), supporting the middle of the face as well as forming the upper jaw.

~~~~~~~~~~

Micronutrients: Nutrients needed by the body but only in small amounts. Micronutrients are measured in micrograms and milligrams and typically include vitamins and minerals.

Vitamin deficiency can be a problem for someone who is not receiving the necessary amounts of a given micronutrient through whole food sources. This was seen in prisoners of war captured by the Japanese during World War II. Since the prisoners were fed plain rice and minimal other nutrients there were many B-vitamin deficiency symptoms among the POWs. Prisoners of war in Europe were usually given potatoes or sweet potatoes as a starch/carbohydrate and this difference prevented a significant amount of vitamin deficiency in the European theater during WWII.

~~~~~~~~~~

Mock-Surgery: A mock-surgery is performed by your surgeon on a model of your upper and lower jaws. The model is created from a mold made when the surgical team makes impressions of your upper and lower teeth to check the alignment. The surgeon takes the models and performs a basic mock-surgery similar to the procedures expected for the patient. This tests the probable results if surgery were performed at this time.

When the mock-surgery yields good results and the surgeon feels that more orthodontic adjustments will likely not improve the patient's potential beyond the current potential results, the patient will be surgery-ready. The surgical team will arrange with the patient for the pre-surgery appointment and testing and set a date for surgery.

~~~~~~~~~~

Occlusion: The occlusion refers to the way in which the upper teeth and lower teeth come together when the mouth closes or bites. Occlusion is basically a fancy word for "alignment" or "bite."

~~~~~~~~~~

Offense: The Offense in football is the active portion of the team that works to score points. In the Jaw Recovery Playbook, the Offense consists primarily of the patient who works as their own Quarterback and Team Captain. The Defense works with the patient to provide support and assistance when needed.

~~~~~~~~~~

Offensive Coordinators: In the Jaw Recovery Playbook, the Offensive Coordinators are the medical professionals providing care and treatment for the patient. This will generally include the orthodontist and surgeon or surgical team.

Although the orthodontist and surgeon(s) are responsible for communicating effectively throughout the care of the patient, this communication is sometimes less-than-efficient. As the Team Captain, the patient should double-check to ensure all members of the team are in sync.

~~~~~~~~~~

Oral & Maxillofacial Surgery: Also referred to as OMFS. A field of medical and/or dental surgery responsible for treating, correcting, improving, or repairing injuries and defects within the realm of the head, face, neck, jaws, tissue (hard and soft) of the mouth, face, and jaws.

Oral & Maxillofacial Surgeons often perform cosmetic procedures such as genioplasty and rhinoplasty, as well as medically necessary, corrective procedures.

Your Oral & Maxillofacial Surgeon may hold a degree in dentistry (DDS or DMD) or a degree in medicine (MD); in the United States, depending on where your surgeon is from (originally and academically), both are recognized as qualified to train and perform surgeries in the OMFS field but many OMF surgeons are Doctors of Dental Surgery.

Orthodontist: Orthodontists are dentists trained and specializing in the straightening or adjusting of teeth to repair or correct malocclusions. The malocclusion may be caused by uneven teeth, disproportion in the upper jaw, lower jaw, or both, and other irregularities that create problems for patients.

Orthognathic Surgery: Orthognathic surgery refers to corrective surgeries performed on the jaws (or face). The surgery may correct an alignment, malformation, or related problems, as well as working to correct deformities such as cleft palate. Orthgnathic surgery is also known as "corrective jaw surgery."

Palate: The roof of the mouth.

PCM: Primary Care Manager; Usually a general doctor that performs the patient's physical exams and treats minor illnesses that do not require a specialist.

PCP: Primary Care Physician; Another term for the PCM or general doctor.

Playbook System: The Jaw Recovery Playbook System is a series of individual Playbooks or "guides" that assist in informing patients of the orthodontic treatment and jaw surgery processes, helping patients' families and loved ones prepare for jaw surgery to better assist the patient, and helping patients and surgeons communicate on a more effective level for greater patient-compliance, better results, and generally better patient satisfaction at the completion of treatment.

The Playbook System consists of the website www.JawRecoveryPlaybook.com as well as the individual Playbooks available separately or as a Playbook Bundle. Visit the website for more details!

Primary Care Manager: The general doctor or primary physician of a patient. Also PCM or PCP.

Primary Care Physician: The general doctor or primary physician of a patient. Also PCP or PCM.

Proxabrush: A special toothbrush designed to fit between teeth, when gaps are present, but often associated with cleaning between the brackets of braces. The cone-shaped brush is available in a variety of sizes to suit different needs and many Proxabrushes come with two ends so you can use two different sized brushes easily.

Proxabrushes and refills are sold with the regular toothbrushes in grocery stores and pharmacies, often in a separate section of the toothbrush aisle along with floss and floss picks, dental wax, and other specialized oral hygiene tools.

Quarterback: The Quarterback in the Jaw Recovery Playbook is the patient. As the Quarterback, the patient is also the Team Captain and thus responsible for keeping the different team components working together effectively.

Recovery: Following jaw surgery, the upper jaw and/or lower jaw requires a minimum 6-12 weeks to recover. This is the time it takes for the cut bone to reach out and fuse to other cut bone, improving blood flow to these regions for better healing.

Resident: The Residents in a teaching hospital are doctors (medical or dental, usually) that have finished the necessary coursework and training but are now working with patients at different levels under the direct supervision of experienced doctors, dentists, and surgeons depending on the field and specialty.

Rhinoplasty: Also called a "nose job" - rhinoplasty includes any surgical procedure meant to correct or improve the look and/or function of the nose. This makes rhinoplasty both corrective and cosmetic, like jaw surgery procedures, determined by the circumstances.

Self-Ligating Braces: Self-ligating braces have a smaller bracket for more free tooth surface which improves cleaning and oral hygiene efforts throughout treatment. The smaller brackets have a latch that closes around the archwires. The innovative style speeds up treatment, sometimes twice as fast which cuts orthodontic treatment time in half. They are usually more expensive than traditional braces but less expensive than "invisible" ceramic braces (prices will vary between location and specialist).

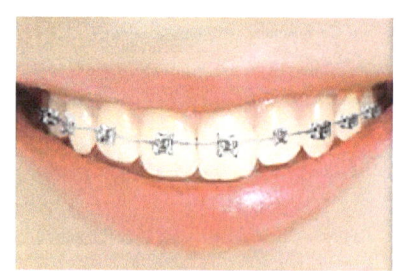

Photo from www.bracesVIP.com

Surgeon: The surgeon is the medical doctor or dentist trained in performing surgical procedures. In this instance, oral & maxillofacial surgeons are trained to perform corrective and cosmetic surgeries for the head, neck, face, and mouth.

Surgical Hooks: Surgical hooks may be attached to the brackets on your teeth or separate elements clamped onto the archwires. There are different styles for different needs. For images and information, visit American Orthodontics (a manufacturer of orthodontics products) at www.americanortho.com/stops-hooks_main.htm

Surgical Team: Your Surgical Team is part of your Offensive Coordinator Team, but generally consists of the Surgeon, any Residents that assist the Surgeon, and also a variety of support staff and technicians including an Anesthesiologist.

During the hospital stay there are other staff and nurses that offer additional support and may be considered part of the extended Surgical Team.

Teaching Hospital: A teaching hospital is a medical facility in which Resident doctors, surgeons, and other medical professionals receive hands-on training supervised by experienced professionals in order to become full-fledged doctors, surgeons, nurses, etc.

Teaching hospitals are often associated with a local medical school or university and are an excellent source of healthcare if you can demonstrate patience as a patient. Teaching hospitals provide specialized medical care and research as well as healthcare for uninsured patients.

When considering a location for jaw surgery, check with local teaching hospitals. They may be easier to work with your budget or your insurance and offer more economical surgery options without compromising quality care.

www.aamc.org/about/teachinghospitals/

Temperomandibular Joint: Often referred to as TMJ, the temporomandibular joint is found at both sides of the jaw when the upper temporal bone meets the mandible. This is a very strong joint in all mammals, associated with the muscles of mastication (chewing) but it is also a common source of pain or problems for some people.

TMJ is NOT the problem, the TMJ is the joint. You have two TMJs. When a problem exists it is referred to as TMD or Temporomandibular Joint Disorder.

Training Camp: Training camp, in football, is just as it sounds. Before the season starts, the different football teams gather at their respective training camps to practice, train, learn, and improve as preparation for the new season.

In the Jaw Recovery Playbook, Training Camp is composed of the individual Playbooks, videos, and other information and resources found at www.JawRecoveryPlaybook.com -- each of which have been tirelessly researched, sorted, written or compiled in an effort to provide jaw surgery patients, their families, orthodontists, and surgeons with quality tools to enhance patient understanding, compliance, and overall treatment and surgery experiences for all involved.

True Lime: A crystalized lime juice from the True Citrus Company. Available in most grocery store chains, you can also purchase True Citrus packets online from www.TrueLemonStore.com I typically mix True Lime (my favorite!) with Truvia (a type of Stevia sweetener) into my water for a subtle-sweetness and a refreshing taste that will not affect blood sugar, hunger, or hydration.

~~~~~~~~~~

Your Team: Your Team is composed of the Quarterback (patient), the Offensive Coordinators (orthodontist, surgeon, surgical team), and the Defense (family, spouse, siblings, children, friends, pets, parents, and anyone offering support or assistance throughout the surgery and recovery process).

The Quarterback is responsible for making sure the Team understands what's going on, managing the appointments, and making sure the surgeon and orthodontist are able to communicate clearly and effectively.

Bibliography & Resources

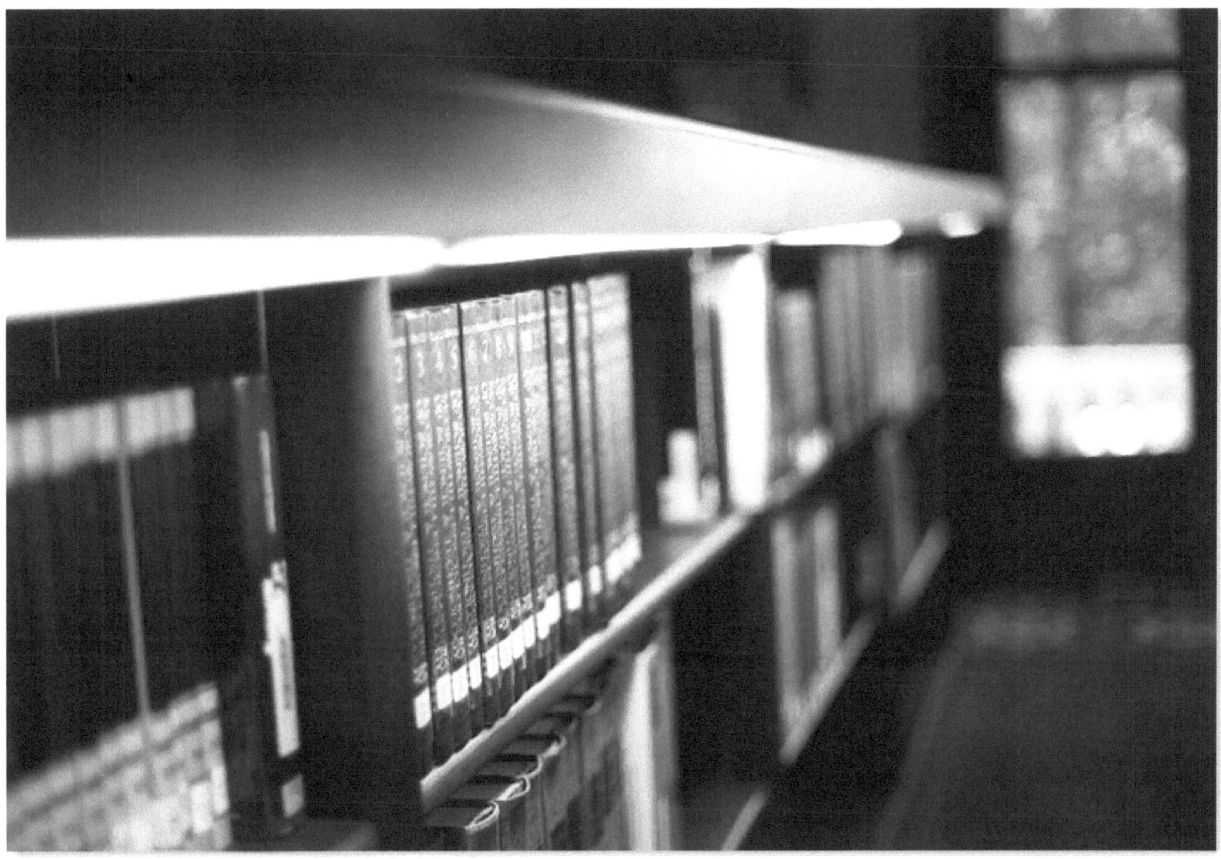

The following bibliography provides a list of the resources I reviewed while studying, researching, and preparing for jaw surgery. To the best of my knowledge, the list is complete, as far as printed resources go. There are so many online resources that just did not provide the type of information I needed to feel comfortable with my understanding of the circumstances so this list of resources is considerably boring (for most people, at least) and it is definitely not for the casual reader. These resources are not cited throughout the text simply because I read and took notes for myself, without the intention of compiling a resource for others. As I read and took notes, the information synthesized naturally for me, allowing me to create the Playbook System with accuracy.

The Jaw Recovery Playbook System intended to be an approachable resource for other jaw surgery patients; not a research project, despite its appearances at times. I did list the resources according to the American Psychological Association (APA) Guidelines because my formal education is in Psychology and that is the format I typically use for research papers.

I chose to include this bibliography to show that the information was not merely from my own experience as a jaw surgery patient, but from scientifically and medically recognized research and educational resources. The Additional References section is mostly non-scholarly resources, thus the separation.

~ Sasha

Adewole, R. A. and Akinwande, J. A. (2007). Public and professional perception of oral and maxillofacial surgery (a pilot study). *Nig Q J Hosp Med, 17(1)*, 8-12. Retrieved from http://www.ncbi.nlm.nih.gov/pubmed/17688165

Akita, K., Shimokawa, T., and Sato, T. (2000). Positional relationships between the masticatory muscles and their innervating nerves with special reference to the lateral pterygoid and the midmedial and discotemporal muscle bundles of temporalis. *Journal of Anaomy, 197*, 291-302. Retrieved from http://onlinelibrary.wiley.com/store/10.1046/j.1469-7580.2000.19720291.x/asset/j.1469-7580.2000.19720291.x.pdf?v=1&t=hcdda07b&s=5e7016eb76521c1f3cd52ad1a649b85452209fa3

Allen, P. J., D'Anci, K. E., Kanarek, R. B., and Renshaw, P. F. (2010). Chronic creatine supplementation alters depression-like behavior in rodents in a sex-dependent manner. *Neuropsychopharmacology, 35*, 534-546. Retrieved from http://www.ncbi.nlm.nih.gov/pmc/articles/PMC2794979/

Attar. B. M. and Far, N. F. (2009). Neurosensory changes of palatal mucousa following Le Fort I osteotomy. *Journal of Research in Medical Sciences, 14(5)*, 269-275. Retrieved from http://www.ncbi.nlm.nih.gov/pmc/articles/PMC3129095/?report=printable

Balaji, S. M. (2010). Change of lip and occlusal cant after simultaneous maxillary and mandibular distraction osteogenesis in hemifacial microsomia. *Journal of Oral and Maxillofacial Surgery, 9(4)*, 344-349. Retrieved from http://www.ncbi.nlm.nih.gov/pmc/articles/PMC3177468/

Bhuvaneswaran, M. (2010). Principles of smile design. *Journal of Conservative Dentistry, 13(4)*, 225-232. Retrieved from http://www.ncbi.nlm.nih.gov/pmc/articles/PMC3010027/?tool=pmcentrez

Brennan, D. S., Singh, K., Spencer, A. J., and Roberts-Thomson, K. F. (2006). Positive and negative affect and oral health-related quality of life. *Health and Quality of Life Outcomes, 4(1)*, 83. Retrieved from http://www.hqlo.com/content/4/1/83

Dujoncquoy, JP., Ferri, J., Raoul, G., and Kleinheinz, J. (2010). Temporomandibular joint dysfunction and orthognathic surgery: A retrospective study. *Head and Face Medicine, 6(1)*, 27. Retrieved from http://www.head-face-med.com/content/6/1/27

Dura, E., Andreu, Y., Galdon, M. J., Ferrando, M., Murgui, S., Poveda, R., and Bagain, J.V. (2006). Psychological assessment of patients with temporomandibular disorders: confirmatory analysis of the dimensional structure of the Brief Symptoms Inventory 18. *International Journal of Psychosomatic Research, 60(4)*, 365-370.

Ferrando, M., Galdon, M. J., Dura, E., Andreu, Y., Jimenex, Y., and Poveda, R. (2012). Enhancing the efficacy of treatment for temporomandibular patients with muscular diagnosis through cognitive-behavioral intervention, including hypnosis: A randomized study. Oral Surgery, Oral Medicine, *Oral Pathology and Oral Radiology, 113(1),* 81-89. Retrieved from http://bscw.rediris.es/pub/bscw.cgi/d4448152/Ferrando-Enhancing_efficacy_treatment_temporomandibular_patients.pdf

Foltan, R. and Sedy, J. (2009). Behavioral changes of patients after orthognathic surgery develop on the basis of the loss of vomeronasal organ: A hypothesis. *Head and Face Medicine, 5(1),* 5. Retrieved from http://www.head-face-med.com/content/5/1/5

Fukuda, K., Hayashida, M., Ikeda, K., Koukita, Y., Ichinohe, T., and Kaneko, Y. ((2010). Diversity of opioid requirements for postoperative pain control following oral surgery 0 Is it affected by polymorphism of the μ-opioid receptor? *Anesthesia Progress, 57,* 145-149. Retrieved from http://www.ncbi.nlm.nih.gov/pmc/articles/PMC3006662/

Forsman, A. (2008). ETSU, Anatomy & Physiology 1 (Lectures). *Apple iTunes U.* Retrieved from https://itunes.apple.com/us/itunes-u/anatomy-physiology-i/id384931539

Forsman, A. (2008). ETSU, Anatomy & Physiology 2 (Lectures). *Apple iTunes U.* Retrieved from https://itunes.apple.com/us/itunes-u/anatomy-physiology-ii/id384931669

Forsman, A. (2008). ETSU, Anatomy & Physiology VidCast – Lab Videos. *Apple iTunes U.* Retrieved from https://itunes.apple.com/us/itunes-u/anatomy-physiology-vidcast/id384931548

Gintaras, J. and Wang, H. (2010). Guidelines for the identification of the mandibular vital structures: Practical clinical applications of anatomy and radiological examination methods. *Journal of Oral and Maxillofacial Research, 2(1),* e1. Retrieved from http://www.ejomr.org/JOMR/archives/2010/2/e1/e1ht.pdf

Hassett, L. C. (1990). Summary of the scientific literature for pain and anxiety control in dentistry [a bibliography]. *Anesthesia Progress, 37,* 208-215.

Hongiman, R. J., Phillips, K. A., and Castle, D. J. (2004) A review of psychosocial outcomes for patients seeking cosmetic surgery. *Plast Reconstr Surg, 113(4),* 1229-1237. Retrieved from http://www.ncbi.nlm.nih.gov/pmc/articles/PMC1762095/

Hunter, M. J., Rubeiz, T., and Rose L. (1996). Recognition of the scope of oral and maxillofacial surgery by the public and health care professionals. *Journal of Oral and Maxillofacial Surgery, 54(10),* 1227-1232. Retrieved from http://www.ncbi.nlm.nih.gov/pubmed/8859242 (excerpt)

Iliopoulos, Ch., Zouloumis, L., Lazaridou, M. (2010). Physiology of bone turnover and its application in contemporary maxillofacial surgery. A review. *HIPPOKRATIA, 14(4)*, 244-248. Retrieved from http://www.ncbi.nlm.nih.gov/pmc/articles/PMC3031317/

Jerjes, W., Upile, T., Kafas, P., Abbas, S., Rob, J., McCarthy, E., McCarthy, P., and Hopper, C. (2009). Debate article; Third molar surgery: The patient's and the clinician's perspective. *International Archives of Medicine, 2(1),* 32. Retrieved from http://www.intarchmed.com/content/2/1/32

Juodzbalys, G., Wang, H., Sabalys, G. (2010). Anatomy of mandibular vital structures. Part I: Mandibular canal and inferior alveolar neurovascular bundle in relation with dental implantology. *Journal of Oral and Maxillofacial Research, 1(1),* e2. Retrieved from http://ejomr.org/JOMR/archives/2010/1/e2/e2ht.pdf

Juodzbalys, G., Wang, H., Sabalys, G. (2010). Anatomy of mandibular vital structures. Part II: Mandibular incisive canal, mental foramen, and associated neurovascular bundles in relation with dental implantology. *Journal of Oral and Maxillofacial Research, 1(1),* e3. Retrieved from http://ejomr.org/JOMR/archives/2010/1/e3/e3ht.pdf

Kafas, P., Upile, T., Angouridakis, N., Stavrianos, C., Dabarakis, N., and Jerjes, W. (2009). Dysaesthesia in the mental nerve distribution triggered by a foreign body: A case report. *Cases Journal, 2(1),* 169. Retrieved from http://www.casesjournal.com/content/2/1/169

Kalm, L. M. and Semba, R. D. (2005). They Starved so that Others be Better Fed: Remembering Ancel Keys and the Minnesota Experiment. *The Journal of Nutrition, 135(6),* 1347-1352. Retreived from http://jn.nutrition.org/content/135/6/1347.full

Landim, F. S., Freitas, G. B., Malouf, A. B., Carvalho Studart, L. P., Rocha, N. S., Andrade, E. S., Caubi, A. F., Rodrigues, J., Filho, L., and Silva, E. D. O. (2011). Repercussions of surgically assisted maxillary expansion on nose width and position of septum and inferior nasal conchae. *International Journal of Medical Sciences, 8(8),* 659-666. Retrieved from http://www.medsci.org/v08p0659.pdf

Mesgarzadeh, A., Motamedi, M. H. K., Akhavan, H., Tousi, T. S., Mehrvarzfar, P., and Eshkevari, P. S. (2010). Effects of Le Fort I osteotomy on maxillary anterior teeth: A 5-year follow up of 42 cases. *Eplasty, 8(10),* e10. Retrieved from https://www.researchgate.net/publication/41103169_Effects_of_Le_Fort_I_osteotomy_on_maxillary_anterior_teeth_a_5-year_follow_up_of_42_cases

Nagatsuke, C., Ichinohe, T., and Kaneko, Y. (2000). Preemptive effects of a combination of preoperative diclofenac, butorphanol, and lidocaine on postoperative pain management following orthognathic surgery. *Anesthesia Progress, 47,* 119-124. Retrieved from http://www.ncbi.nlm.nih.gov/pmc/articles/PMC2149035/pdf/anesthprog00224-0007.pdf

Phillips, C. and Blakey III, G. (2008). Short-term recovery after orthognathic surgery: A medical daily diary approach. *International Journal of Oral and Maxillofacial Surgery, 37(10),* 892-896. Retrieved from http://pubmedcentralcanada.ca/pmcc/articles/PMC2590780/pdf/nihms79857.pdf

Phillips, C., Blakey III, G., and Essick, G. K. (2011). Sensory retraining: A cognitive behavioral therapy for altered sensation. *Atlas Oral Maxillofac Surg Clin North Am., 19(1),* 109-118. Retrieved from http://www.ncbi.nlm.nih.gov/pmc/articles/PMC3073500/pdf/nihms253811.pdf

Phillips, C., Blakey III, G., and Jaskolka, M. (2008). Recovery after orthognathic surgery: Short-term health-related quality of life outcomes. *Journal of Oral and Maxillofacial Surgery, 66(10),* 2110-2115. Retrieved from http://www.ncbi.nlm.nih.gov/pmc/articles/PMC2585944/

Phillips, C., Essick, G., Zuniga, J., Tucker, M., Blakey III, G. (2006). Qualitative descriptors used by patients following orthognathic surgery to portray altered sensation. *Journal of Oral and Maxillofacial Surgery, 64(12),* 1751-1760. Retrieved from http://www.ncbi.nlm.nih.gov/pmc/articles/PMC2869201/

Phillips, C., Kim, S. H., Tucker, M., and Turvey, T. A. (2010). Sensory retraining: Burden in daily life related to altered sensation after orthognathic surgery, a randomized clinical trial. *Orthodontics and Craniofacial Research, 13(3),* 169-178. Retrieved from http://www.ncbi.nlm.nih.gov/pmc/articles/PMC2904648/

Roitman, S., Green, T., Osher, Y., Karni, N., and Levine, J. (2007). Creatine monohydrate in resistant depression: A preliminary study. *Bipolar Disorders, 9(7),* 754-758. Retrieved from http://www.joseph-levine.co.il/wp-content/uploads/2009/01/creatine-depression.pdf

Rustemeyer, J., Eke, Z., Bremerich, A. (2010). Perception of improvement after orthognathic surgery: The important variables affecting patient satisfaction. *Oral and Maxillofacial Surgery, 14(3),* 155-162. Retrieved from http://www.ncbi.nlm.nih.gov/pmc/articles/PMC2928919/

Said Yekta, S., Koch, F., Grosjean, M. B., Esteves-Oliveira, M., Stein, J. M., Ghassemi, A., Riediger, D., Lampert, F., Smeets, R. (2010). Analysis of trigeminal nerve disorders after oral and maxillofacial intervention. *Head & Face Medicine, 6(1),* 24. Retrieved from http://www.head-face-med.com/content/6/1/24

Scientific Publishing, Ltd. (2010). Anatomy & Physiology Flash Cards. Illinois: *Scientific Publishing, Ltd.*

Smolin, L. A. and Grosvenor, M. B. (2003). Nutrition: Science and Application, Fourth Edition. *John Wiley & Sons, Inc.*

Torii, K. and Chiwata, I. (2007). Occlusal management for a patient with aural symptoms of unknown etiology: a case report. *Journal of Medical Case Reports, 1(1),* 85. Retrieved from http://www.ncbi.nlm.nih.gov/pmc/articles/PMC2008203/

Tucker, T. (2006). The Great Starvation Experiment: Ancel Keys and the Men Who Starved for Science. *University of Minnesota Press.*

White, T. D. and Folkens, P. A. (2005). The Human Bone Manual. Elsevier, Inc. *Academic Press.*

Wolford, L. M., Stevao, E. L. L. (2003). Considerations in nerve repair. *Baylor University Medical Center Proceedings, 16,* 152-156. Retrieved from http://www.ncbi.nlm.nih.gov/pmc/articles/PMC1201001/

Additional References (non-scholarly):

8-West Cosmetic Surgery: The Geometry of Beauty http://dev.farfromfearless.com/koz-00003-dev/knowledge-base/reshape/face/the-geometry-of-beauty/

180DegreeHealth.com: Ancel Keys and the Biology of Human Starvation http://180degreehealth.com/2010/03/ancel-keys-and-the-biology-of-human-starvation

American Association of Oral and Maxillofacial Surgeons: Corrective Jaw Surgery http://www.aaoms.org/jaw_surgery.php and Nutrition http://www.aaoms.org/nutrition.php

American Association of Oral and Maxillofacial Surgeons: The Temporomandibular Joint (TMJ) http://www.aaoms.org/tmj.php

American Psychological Association – Plastic Surgery: Beauty or Beast? By Melissa Dittmann http://www.apa.org/monitor/sep05/surgery.aspx

Anesthesiology Info: How Does Anesthesia Work? http://anesthesiologyinfo.com/articles/01062002.php

AshevilleList.com: Conditions in Japanese Prisoner of War Camps in World War II http://www.ashevillelist.com/history/prisoners-wwii.htm

Bartleby.com: The Facial Nerves (from Anatomy of the Human Body by Henry Gray) http://www.bartleby.com/107/202.html

Bone and Spine: How Does Bone Fracture Healing Occur? http://boneandspine.com/trauma/bone-fracture-healing-occur/

British Dental Journal: The Psychology of Dental Patient Care: An Introduction by Elinor Parker http://www.nature.com/bdj/journal/v186/n9/full/4800137a1.html

Captain George Steiger: A POW Diary – Fsteiger.com http://www.fsteiger.com/gsteipow.html

Chronic psychological symptoms in surgical patients Medical University of Berlin http://www.charite.de/en/charite/press/press_reports/artikel/detail/chronische_psychische_beschwerden_bei_operativen_patienten/

The Cleveland Clinic, Center for Continuing Education www.clevelandclinicmeded.com

CNN Health: Not everyone's a good plastic surgery candidate by Linda Saether http://articles.cnn.com/2007-11-30/health/hfh.no.plastic.surgery_1_cosmetic-surgery-plastic-surgery-plastic-surgeons/2?_s=PM:HEALTH

The Dana Foundation: Protecting the Brain from a Glutamate Storm by Vivian Teichberg and Luba Vikhanski http://www.dana.org/news/cerebrum/detail.aspx?id=7376

Dental Lab Direct www.dental-lab-direct.com

Does surgery make a broken bone heal faster? By Jonathen Cluett, M.D. http://orthopedics.about.com/od/castsfracturetreatments/f/faster.htm

Evolutionary Psychiatry Blog by Emily Deans: Semi-Starvation Experiment in Arizona – Biosphere 2 http://evolutionarypsychiatry.blogspot.com/2010/10/semi-starvation-experiment-in-arizona.html

Evolutionary Psychiatry Blog by Emily Deans: Semistarvation Experiments in WWII http://evolutionarypsychiatry.blogspot.com/2010/07/semistarvation-experiments-in-wwii.html

Evolutionary Psychiatry Blog by Emily Deans: Diet, Depression, and Anxiety http://evolutionarypsychiatry.blogspot.com/2010/06/diet-depression-and-anxiety.html

Evolutionary Psychiatry Blog by Emily Deans: Diet and Depression Again http://evolutionarypsychiatry.blogspot.com/2010/06/diet-and-depression-again.html

Face Center Los Angeles (YouTube): Orthognathic (Jaw) Surgery Procedures - a series of short animations demonstrating the different types of jaw surgery http://www.youtube.com/playlist?list=PL9801198906917C87

Fallon Oral Surgery of Syracuse: Home Care http://www.fallonoralsurgery.com/Home-Care.aspx

Family Doctor: Kids – The Facts About Broken Bones http://kidshealth.org/PageManager.jsp?dn=familydoctor&lic=44&cat_id=113&article_set=10508#

Garai Orthodontic Specialists, Vienna, VA. www.bracesvip.com

The Guardian UK: Plastic surgeons issued with psychological checklist by David Batty http://www.guardian.co.uk/society/2006/sep/22/health.medicineandhealth1

Heather's Speech Therapy: Correcting a Frontal Lisp http://heatherspeechtherapy.com/2011/05/correcting-a-frontal-lisp/

How do broken bones heal? By Robert Lamb http://science.howstuffworks.com/life/human-biology/heal-broken-bones2.htm

A Human Face: Facial Nerve http://face-and-emotion.com/dataface/anatomy/peripheralnerves.jsp

A Human Face: Trigeminal Nerve http://face-and-emotion.com/dataface/anatomy/trigeminal.jsp

Inner Body: Nerves of the Head and Neck http://www.innerbody.com/image/nerv01.html

LiveStrong.com: Do Potato Skins Contain Fiber? By Sandy Keefe http://www.livestrong.com/article/343657-do-potato-skins-contain-fiber/

LymphNotes.com: The Lymphatic systemhttp://www.lymphnotes.com/article.php/id/151/

Maine Organic Farmers and Gardeners Association: Potatoes and POWs: How Spuds Saved American GIs in Nazi Prison Camps During World War II by John Koster http://www.mofga.org/Publications/MaineOrganicFarmerGardener/Fall2010/Potatoes/tabid/1726/Default.aspx

MedScape Reference: Psychological Aspects of Plastic Surgery http://emedicine.medscape.com/article/838030-overview

Medscape Reference: Facial Bone Anatomy http://emedicine.medscape.com/article/835401-overview#a1

MedScape Reference: Lips and Perioral Region Anatomy http://emedicine.medscape.com/article/835209-overview#a30

Mendeley: The effects of BOTOX injections on emotional experience by Joshua Ian Davis, Ann Senghas, Fredric Brandt, and Kevin N Ochsner http://www.ncbi.nlm.nih.gov/pmc/articles/PMC2880828/

Michigan Oral Surgeons: Home Care Instructions for Jaw Surgery Patients http://www.michiganoralsurgeons.com/surgical_instruction/after_jaw_surgery.html

Microsoft Office Images and ClipArt www.office.microsoft.com/en-us/images

Minnesota State University: A Collection of Approaches to the "s" Sound by Judy Kuster http://www.mnsu.edu/comdis/kuster2/therapy/stherapy.html

The National Center for Aesthetic Facial and Oral Surgery: Cosmetic Jaw Surgery http://www.maxfac.com/facial/jaw.html

National Institute on Deafness and Other Communication Disorders: Voice, Speech, and Language http://www.nidcd.nih.gov/health/voice/Pages/Default.aspx

The New York Times: Health – Psychology; Emotional preparation aids surgical recovery by Daniel Goleman http://www.nytimes.com/1987/12/10/us/health-psychology-emotional-preparation-aids-surgical-recovery.html

The Orthodontic CYBERJournal: A Patient's Guide to Orthognathic Surgery by Dr. David Darver http://orthocj.com/2000/06/a-patients-guide-to-orthognathic-surgery/

Pearson Assessments: Brief Symptom Inventory – BSI http://psychcorp.pearsonassessments.com/HAIWEB/Cultures/en-us/Productdetail.htm?Pid=PAbsi

Pearson Assessments: Brief Symptom Inventory 18 – BSI 18 http://psychcorp.pearsonassessments.com/HAIWEB/Cultures/en-us/Productdetail.htm?Pid=PAg110

Pearson Assessments: MBMD – Millon Behavioral Medicine Diagnostic http://www.pearsonassessments.com/HAIWEB/Cultures/en-us/Productdetail.htm?Pid=PAg503

Pearson: MBMD Test – Moving from Failure to Success: The MBMD Test Benefits Bariatric Surgeons and Their Patients http://www.pearsonassessments.com/NR/rdonlyres/3EA3E17E-4D93-4A60-9B83-B9CA278E7EAE/0/ProFiles_MBMD_Benefits.pdf

Pearson: Medically oriented psychological tests help improve care for breast surgery candidates http://www.pearsonassessments.com/NR/rdonlyres/69DCA659-1B93-432F-B2FD-7154EEDA5E42/4355/_BTG_Sept07p2.pdf

Pearson: Psychological tests serve as practical teaching tools with advanced psychology students http://www.pearsonassessments.com/NR/rdonlyres/69DCA659-1B93-432F-B2FD-7154EEDA5E42/4278/_BTG_Nov08P2.pdf

Pearson: Psychologist calls MBMD Test key to efficacy and effectiveness http://www.pearsonassessments.com/NR/rdonlyres/69DCA659-1B93-432F-B2FD-7154EEDA5E42/4670/BTG_Fall06p2.pdf

ProteinPower.com – The Blog of Michael R. Eades, M.D.: Is a calorie always a calorie? http://www.proteinpower.com/drmike/metabolism/is-a-calorie-always-a-calorie/

Psychology of the surgical patient by Alexander Kennedy http://www.ncbi.nlm.nih.gov/pmc/articles/PMC2036905/

Rhinoplasty Online: The Best Nose Visualizers on the Internet http://www.rhinoplastyonline.com/best-nose-visualizer.html

Right Track Reading: Addressing Speech Difficulties During Reading Instruction – Tips for Helping a Child Pronounce Specific Sounds http://www.righttrackreading.com/tipstosaysounds.html

SELF – Nutritional Data: Sweet Potato http://nutritiondata.self.com/facts/vegetables-and-vegetable-products/2667/2

Soul Spring Counseling: Benefits of Psychological Preparation for Surgery http://www.soulspringcounselling.com/surgery.htm

Speechlanguage-Resources.com: Speech Sounds S: How to Stimulate the /s/ Sound http://www.speechlanguage-resources.com/speech-sounds-s.html

SpeechPathology.com: Remediation Tongue Thrust by Michelle Harmon, PhD, CCC-SLP http://www.speechpathology.com/ask-the-experts/writing-the-ultimate-hurdle-882

Suggestions for the Pre-Surgical Psychological Assessment of Bariatric Surgery Candidates – Allied Health Sciences Section Ad Hoc Behavioral Health Committee http://s3.amazonaws.com/publicASMBS/GuidelinesStatements/Guidelines/PsychPreSurgicalAssessment.pdf

Tongue thrust: How to fix a tongue thrust by Matthew Curry http://dentistry.helium.com/how-to/10126-how-to-fix-a-tongue-thrust

UCLA Dentistry: Oral Radiology Study Guide http://www.dentistry.ucla.edu/oradguide/index.html

University of Colorado, Muscles "cheat sheet" by Laurie Boriskie http://www.colorado.edu/intphys/iphy3415/Muscles_OIA_LaurieBoriskie.pdf

U.S. Department of health and Human Services Office on Women's Health: Anemia Fact Sheet http://womenshealth.gov/publications/our-publications/fact-sheet/anemia.cfm

Walter Reed National Military Medical Center, Bethesda, MD. www.wrnmmc.capmed.mil

WebMD: Understanding Anemia http://www.webmd.com/a-to-z-guides/understanding-anemia-basics

WiseGEEK.com: What is the Connection Between Anemia and Nausea? http://www.wisegeek.com/what-is-the-connection-between-anemia-and-nausea.htm

Yale University School of Medicine: Cranial Nerves http://www.yale.edu/cnerves/

~~~~~~~~~

My blog www.SashaMaggio.com -- where I left my notes throughout my recovery to help guide the Jaw Recovery Playbook System development.

My YouTube Channel - Jaw Surgery & Recovery Playlist http://www.youtube.com/playlist?list=PLF77223C6BD0A0A7F

The Jaw Recovery Playbook www.JawRecoveryPlaybook.com

www.ingramcontent.com/pod-product-compliance
Lightning Source LLC
Chambersburg PA
CBHW050725180526
45159CB00003B/1131